CONTENTS

INTRODUCTION

Living with a chronic illness and having to deal with annoying symptoms every day is one of the most challenging things a person can go through. And as someone who suffered from gastritis for over five years, I know how difficult it is to live with this disease and to have to endure, every day, the annoying and unbearable symptoms that it causes.

Before I healed my gastritis, I visited many gastroenterologists and spent thousands of dollars on medical tests and procedures, blood tests, and therapies that were useless. Not to mention all the medications that were prescribed to me, which also didn't help me at all. Many of them made me feel worse than I already did.

It was really frustrating every time my doctor performed an expensive test or procedure on me and I heard him say that everything was fine and that nothing wrong was found in that test or procedure. All that plus the side effects that some medications caused me made me feel depressed and hopeless about one day feeling well again or being a normal person.

I was tired of suffering from gastritis; tired of having to inhibit myself from doing things, such as going out with friends or family for fear of eating or drinking something that would cause me a gastritis attack; and tired of having to visit a new gastroenterologist every so often, just to hear him say the same things as the previous ones and to prescribe me the same useless medications. I was simply sick of being sick.

I'm sure you know what it feels like to go through that, having to avoid so many things that you would like to do, being unable to eat or drink what you want, feeling that nobody can help you solve your health problems—and, worse yet, that people around you (friends, family, and even your doctor) believe that it is all in your head. It is really depressing.

And it was exactly all that which made me, one day, decide to take my health in my hands and do things on my own. I stopped hoping to find someone who would help me regain my health and I stopped looking for that miraculous pill or supplement that would cure all my stomach problems. Instead, I began to research gastritis day and night—what causes it, why it is difficult to cure it, and what I had to do (including how and in what order) to end this nightmare.

It took me five years and thousands of hours spent reading medical and scientific research, articles on blogs and websites, and dozens of healing success stories on online health forums to understand every aspect of this disease and to find a treatment that not only worked for me, but that could also work for anyone who suffers from this disease. And that is what I am going to share with you in this book.

The Gastritis Healing Book is more than just a book about gastritis. It is a comprehensive guide that offers a completely new treatment approach that incorporates precise advice and recommendations about the changes you should make in your diet, habits, and lifestyle, in order to heal your stomach.

This book is divided into three parts:

In the first part, you will learn exactly what gastritis is, what types of gastritis exist, how and why it occurs, what symptoms it causes, and how it is diagnosed. Apart from that, you will learn why it is difficult to cure gastritis (especially chronic cases, which are the ones that last the longest) and what factors may be preventing your stomach from recovering.

In the second part, we will talk about the healing program, which consists of three main steps.

There, I will give you precise advice and recommendations about all the foods that you should either eliminate and introduce into your diet, which bad eating habits can most affect your stomach lining (and that you should eliminate), and which changes you must make in your lifestyle to facilitate the recovery of your stomach. This part also includes a list of supplements and natural remedies that will help you speed up the recovery process of your stomach lining.

In the third part, you will find a one-week meal plan and more than 50 gluten-free and dairy-free recipes, which were carefully developed to make sure they are gastritis-friendly. Both the meal plan and the recipes are included to make it easier for you to follow the diet for gastritis that we will talk about in this book.

In the appendices at the end of the book, I have included useful tips and recommendations that can be very helpful for you. In Appendix A, I talk about some things you can do to recover faster from a flare-up. In Appendix B, I give useful advice on how to stop taking antacid medications such as the popular proton pump inhibitors (PPIs). In Appendix C, I talk about what you can do to gain weight in case you have lost a lot of weight due to gastritis.

What really makes this book unique and different is that most of the information in it is based on scientific evidence rather than someone's opinion. Throughout the text, you will find superscript numbers that relate to citations of the study or research that is the source of the provided information. All scientific studies and research are mentioned in the references at the end of the book; you can easily locate them using the citation number.

I sincerely hope that this book is the solution that you have been seeking and that this is your first step toward a happier, pain-free, and gastritis-free life.

CHAPTER 1:WHAT IS GASTRITIS?

Gastritis is nothing more than the inflammation of the stomach lining, also known as the gastric mucosa, which is the layer that lines the inner layers (submucosa, muscularis, and serosa) of the stomach, and which, in turn, is covered by another layer that protects it from irritating substances such as stomach acid and pepsin.

The layer that protects the stomach lining is known as the mucosal barrier and is composed mainly of gastric mucus and bicarbonate. Gastritis usually appears when the existing balance of the mucosal barrier is broken. This allows stomach acid and other substances to irritate and inflame the stomach lining.

The gastric glands are found in the stomach lining. These glands are formed by several types of cells that secrete different substances. Some of the cells found in the gastric glands are as follows: parietal cells that secrete hydrochloric or stomach acid, a substance that gives a low pH range to gastric juices; the chief cells that secrete pepsinogen, which is the precursor to the enzyme pepsin and which, in its active form, helps break down the proteins found in food; and superficial epithelial cells, which produce a thin adherent layer of protective mucus to prevent stomach acid and pepsin from digesting the gastric mucosa and stomach walls. In addition, these superficial epithelial cells secrete bicarbonate, which accumulates in the mucosal barrier and significantly weakens the acidity of gastric juices.

Types of Gastritis and Causes

There are different types of gastritis as well as many possible causes for each of them. However, in general, gastritis can be classified as either acute or chronic. In addition, it can be subdivided into erosive, non-erosive, hemorrhagic, and viral, among others. Next, we will talk about the most common types of gastritis and their causes, to help you understand the differences between each of them.

Acute Gastritis

Acute gastritis is one of the most common types of gastritis and is characterized by a superficial or deep inflammation of the stomach lining that occurs quickly and unexpectedly. The inflammation can be mild, moderate, or severe, although it usually occurs more regularly in deep form accompanied by hemorrhages.

It is important to note that the term "acute" does not refer to the severity of gastritis but, rather, indicates the time of evolution. Therefore, in acute gastritis, the time of evolution is well-defined and the specific onset of the condition is known. In most cases, acute gastritis is a transient episode. However, if this type of gastritis is not properly treated or if those who suffer from it do not receive the appropriate treatment, it can become chronic gastritis with the passage of time.

The causes of acute gastritis are multiple but it is important to know them all as much as possible, as the correct treatment can depend a lot on the underlying cause (regardless of whether it is acute or chronic gastritis).

Most common causes of acute gastritis:

• **Nonsteroidal Anti-Inflammatory Drugs (NSAIDs):** Certain medications such as ibuprofen, diclofenac, and naproxen (including salicylic acid, commonly known as aspirin) damage the stomach mucosa and inhibit the synthesis of prostaglandins, which are responsible for regulating the production of gastric mucus and bicarbonate. Without enough prostaglandins, the stomach lining cannot protect itself from stomach acid and other irritating substances, which makes the stomach more susceptible to suffering some kind of damage.[1]

- **Helicobacter pylori:** One of the most common causes of gastritis and gastroduodenal ulcers in the world is the H. pylori infection. It is estimated that over 50% of the world's population is infected by this bacteria, which can live in the stomach lining without causing problems. However, while most infected people do not have symptoms, in some cases, H. pylori can cause acute gastritis and gastroduodenal ulcers. This bacteria is transmitted through saliva, vomiting, feces, and drinking water or contaminated food.[2]
- **Alcohol:** Excessive alcohol consumption is another very common cause of gastritis. In this case, it is known as alcoholic gastritis. Alcohol is considered one of the most aggressive drinks for the stomach because it wears the mucosal barrier, inflames the stomach walls, and can potentially lead to the appearance of atrophic gastritis and bleeding in the stomach lining.[3,4] Consequently, when the mucosal barrier wears down, the stomach walls are exposed to more stomach acid and other irritating substances, allowing them to cause more damage and inflammation in the stomach.

Other, less common causes are:
- The intake of corrosive or caustic substances such as bleach, strong acids, or poison.[5]
- Viral infections caused by viruses such as cytomegalovirus and Epstein-Barr (especially in people with a weak immune system).[6,7]
- Smoking and recreational drug use.[8]

Acute gastritis can also be a consequence of an acute stress reaction, which often manifests as erosive acute gastritis.[9] The acute stress reaction, also called acute stress disorder or psychological shock, is a condition that arises in response to a scary or traumatic event that induces a strong emotional response in those who experience it. This type of stress gastritis is related to a decrease in blood flow to the stomach and a deterioration in the ability of the stomach lining to protect and renew itself.

Chronic Gastritis

This type of gastritis is characterized by the progressive inflammation of the stomach lining over time. The main difference between chronic and acute gastritis is its time of onset, as acute gastritis suddenly arises but its symptoms usually disappear as the condition improves. The term "chronic," on the other hand, refers to the fact that it is a problem that is deeply rooted or that has long been in existence. However, "chronic" does not mean that it is incurable.

Unlike with acute gastritis, many people who suffer from chronic gastritis do not experience any symptoms or discomfort during the first months of the disease, and may even become completely asymptomatic. Most often, this is seen in cases of mild or inactive superficial chronic gastritis. Still, no matter what type of gastritis it is, it should be treated to avoid future complications such as gastric ulcers or other, more serious complications.

The causes of chronic gastritis are almost always the same as those that cause the appearance of acute gastritis, with the only difference being that we are faced with causes that last longer.

Most common causes of chronic gastritis:
- **Stress:** When you are stressed, gastric secretions decrease, including the production of gastric mucus and bicarbonate. This, in turn, leaves the stomach lining prone to stomach acid and other substances that can irritate it more easily.[10] However, when stress is constant and prolonged, it can lead to the appearance of chronic gastritis, which, at the least expected time, can begin to cause discomfort and a multitude of symptoms.

- **Helicobacter pylori:** It is estimated that between 60-80% of cases of chronic gastritis are related to a coexisting infection by H. pylori.[11] In most cases, chronic gastritis by H. pylori is due to the fact that during the early phase of the infection, this bacteria causes an acute inflammatory response that is usually asymptomatic and goes unnoticed.[12] This prevents it from being treated at the time it begins to inflame and colonize the stomach lining.
- **Alcohol:** Regular consumption of alcoholic beverages may lead to the appearance of chronic gastritis over time because the constant presence of alcohol in the stomach keeps the stomach lining inflamed and prevents it from recovering and renewing itself.
- **Nonsteroidal anti-inflammatory drugs (NSAIDs):** Excessive use of this type of medication (ibuprofen, naproxen, diclofenac, aspirin, etc.) may cause acute gastritis at first and, over time, prevail as the initial cause of your chronic gastritis if it is not properly treated in its acute phase.
- **Low levels of stomach acid:** One cause of gastritis that is often overlooked is low stomach acid, also known as hypochlorhydria. In itself, the production of gastric mucus is proportional to the amount of acid that your stomach produces. Thus, when your stomach produces little acid, the food spends more time inside it. This allows the acid and other substances to irritate and inflame the stomach lining. Low stomach acid can be caused by different factors, among which are chronic stress, antacid medications, H. pylori infection, zinc deficiency, among others.

Other, less common causes are:
- Alkaline or duodenogastric reflux, which is nothing more than the reflux of bile and pancreatic juices from the small intestine into the stomach.[13] The main irritants contained in bile and pancreatic juices are protease enzyme and bile acids, which destroy the gastric mucus and inflame the stomach lining.
- Certain digestive disorders—such as Crohn's disease—that inflame the gastrointestinal tract.[14]
- A malfunction of the immune system that causes an inflammation of the stomach lining, which, in turn, affects and degrades the stomach cells. This is also known as a type A autoimmune gastritis and is one of the less common causes of chronic gastritis.[15]

The reason why some of the causes of acute gastritis can also cause chronic gastritis is that it is difficult to regain the balance between the protection and repair of the stomach once the stomach lining loses its integrity. This is due to the fact that substances such as stomach acid and pepsin constantly irritate the stomach lining, preventing the restoration of the balance between the protection and repair of the stomach.

That said, it is important to note that, most often, gastritis is usually multifactorial—that is, it is caused by multiple factors that affect the stomach lining. For example, keeping the body under a state of constant stress, eating poorly, and drinking alcohol or taking NSAIDs can create the perfect environment for the appearance of gastritis.

On the other hand, regardless of whether gastritis is chronic or acute, it can be classified as "erosive" or "non-erosive". When it is "erosive," small lesions (superficial tears) appear that can wear the stomach lining and cause stomach ulcers. Meanwhile, when gastritis is "non-erosive," there is only inflammation in the stomach; ulcer formation is not promoted.

Less Common Gastritis

Apart from acute and chronic gastritis, there are other types of gastritis that are usually uncommon and that each has a different cause. However, while it is true that the following types of gastritis are not usually common, they are also classified as acute or chronic. Let's look at the less frequent types of gastritis and the difference between each of them.

• **Hemorrhagic gastritis:** This is a condition in which, due to superficial erosions of the stomach lining, the stomach begins to bleed. The most frequent cause of this type of gastritis is the consumption of acetylsalicylic acid (aspirin), non-steroidal anti-inflammatory drugs, and alcohol.[16]

• **Atrophic gastritis:** This type of gastritis is mainly characterized by atrophy or the gradual loss of gastric cells. There are two types of chronic atrophic gastritis, which are autoimmune gastritis and multifocal gastritis. In autoimmune gastritis, the immune system (antibodies) attacks stomach cells, especially parietal cells, which, apart from producing stomach acid, also produce intrinsic factor. The intrinsic factor is a glycoprotein that helps absorb vitamin B12 in the intestines. On the other hand, chronic multifocal atrophic gastritis is a type of gastritis that is commonly observed in the antrum and body of the stomach. It is caused mainly by the infection of the bacteria Helicobacter pylori.[17]

• **Phlegmonous gastritis:** This type of acute gastritis is a fairly rare but potentially dangerous form, characterized by suppurative inflammation and damage to the stomach wall. People with a weakened immune system are more likely to suffer from this type of gastritis. The main cause of this condition is an infection by pyogenic bacteria that produces pus in the stomach.[18]

• **Lymphocytic gastritis:** This is a type of chronic gastritis that usually affects the antral area of the stomach and is characterized by the presence of lymphocytes that form nodules and complete follicles. Lymphocytic gastritis may not present an apparent cause; in fact, in most cases, it is idiopathic (of unknown cause). However, some studies confirm that a percentage of this gastritis is caused by the presence of the bacteria Helicobacter pylori.[19,20]

• **Granulomatous gastritis:** This is a type of gastritis that consists of chronic inflammation of the stomach lining but of a granulomatous type. Usually, this type of gastritis does not occur on its own but co-occurs with systemic diseases such as tuberculosis, sarcoidosis, syphilis, or Crohn's disease. Despite not having a specific area of affection, it is located more frequently in the antral area of the stomach.[21]

• **Eosinophilic gastritis:** This is another rare type of gastritis that affects predominantly the stomach and small intestine. It is classified as nonspecific, with abundant eosinophils (white blood cells) observed in the gastric mucosa, and can spread to the serosa and muscularis layer of the stomach. The causes of this peculiar condition are still unknown but sometimes there is a related allergic disease or the presence of parasites.[22]

Apart from the types of gastritis mentioned above, other related terms can be found, which refer to the classification according to the part of the stomach where the inflammation occurs.

When the inflammatory process is located in the stomach antrum, it is known as antral gastritis, while if the affected area turns out to be the fundus or body of the stomach, it is a fundal or body gastritis. However, when inflammation is present throughout the stomach (fundus, body, antrum, etc.), it is known as pangastritis. After all, the most common thing among all types of gastritis that exist is the inflammation and damage of the stomach lining.

Symptoms of Gastritis

Some people who suffer from certain types of gastritis may not experience any symptoms, so they are considered asymptomatic. However, most people who suffer from gastritis do experience symptoms, which usually vary from one person to another. The most common symptoms of gastritis are the following:

- Stomach pain
- Heartburn or acid reflux
- Nausea or upset stomach
- Vomiting
- Loss of appetite
- Fatigue or tiredness
- Indigestion or stomach heaviness
- Abdominal swelling
- Diarrhea
- Belching and gas
- Loose or dark stools
- Dizziness or feeling faint
- Breathing problems
- Chest pain
- Weight loss

Gastritis affects those who suffer from it differently. The symptoms that a particular person may present often do not coincide with the symptoms that others have, even if the individuals suffer from the same type of gastritis. Let's talk a bit more about the symptoms we have mentioned above so that you can learn more about the way they affect you and present themselves.

- **Stomach pain:** Inflammation of the stomach lining can cause stomach pain, which is sometimes perceived as discomfort in the upper abdomen.[23] This pain or discomfort can appear at any time of the day but it usually appears after eating.

- **Heartburn or acid reflux:** It is common for most people with gastritis to feel heartburn or acid reflux. That burning sensation can be very annoying and can occur at any time of the day.

- **Nausea or upset stomach:** People who suffer from gastritis often feel the sensation of vomiting, especially in the first months of illness and when they have flare-ups. That feeling of wanting to vomit is nothing more than nausea, which can even cause vomiting in those who experience it. In most cases, nausea is the result of stomach irritation.[23]

- **Vomiting:** It is possible that due to the severe inflammation or irritation in the stomach, you want to expel all the content of your stomach outward. This is usually common if you suffer from severe gastritis. Vomiting is a natural reflex that often occurs as a form of protection.

- **Loss of appetite:** It is common to have a loss of appetite when some of the symptoms mentioned above are present. The body can react in this way when the stomach is very irritated and inflamed.

- **Fatigue:** This symptom can have different causes, including adrenal fatigue and inflammation or irritation in the stomach.[23] When it is caused by adrenal fatigue, constant stress (physical or emotional) depletes the reserves of cortisol of the adrenal glands, which makes you feel extreme tiredness, exhaustion, or weakness.

- **Indigestion or stomach heaviness:** This is a common symptom that occurs during, immediately after, or hours after eating. Indigestion can get worse when you are under a situation of constant stress.
- **Abdominal swelling:** Many people who suffer from gastritis experience symptoms like abdominal swelling, which often causes cramps or pain in the intestine. This symptom can be caused mainly by poorly digested foods that pass into the intestine.
- **Diarrhea:** Most of the time, diarrhea is due to poor absorption of fats, though it can also be caused by food intolerances (for example, lactose), poorly digested food that passes into the intestine, and an imbalance in the gut flora.
- **Belching and gas:** Indigestion of food often causes belching and gas in the intestines. Both symptoms usually appear hours after eating.
- **Loose or dark stools:** It is common that, due to poor digestion of food, feces have a loose consistency and a yellowish color. If you are suffering from hemorrhagic gastritis, it is also possible that the stool becomes dark due to internal bleeding.
- **Dizziness or faint feeling:** This is another symptom that occurs frequently and is most often due to severe stomach irritation and inflammation. This symptom can be very annoying and can make everyday tasks more difficult.
- **Breathing problems:** Some people who suffer from gastritis may feel that they are short of breath or cannot breathe properly. This symptom is often due to the acid that rises into the esophagus and that irritates the airways and larynx, causing respiratory problems.
- **Chest pain:** This is a rare symptom that is usually experienced in the form of a small "stabbing" in the chest. It may be related to acid reflux.
- **Weight loss:** Another very common symptom of gastritis is weight loss, which is most often due to a deficiency of stomach acid or digestive enzymes, the poor absorption of food, or not eating the number of calories that your body needs to maintain its weight.

Most of the previously mentioned symptoms can occur regardless of the type of gastritis from which you suffer. This list includes only the symptoms that occur most frequently when one is suffering from gastritis. Thus, it is possible that some people have other nonspecific symptoms not included in the above list.

How is Gastritis Diagnosed?

The diagnosis of gastritis is established by a complete medical history and examination of the patient's stomach. Usually, when the symptoms or signs of digestive problems are present, the attending physician is the one who refers the patient to a gastroenterologist, who is a specialist in diseases of the digestive system. The gastroenterologist interviews the patient to learn more about his symptoms, medical history, lifestyle, and any medication he or she is taking. Once the specialist has collected all that information, he or she determines what tests should be performed. These may include complementary tests to identify other possible causes of non-specific symptoms that the patient may be experiencing.

The definitive diagnosis of gastritis is established by endoscopy or gastroscopy, which is a test aimed at discovering injuries and looking for signs of inflammation in the stomach or of other diseases of greater relevance. The endoscope is also used to examine the lining of the esophagus and the first portion of the small intestine. In addition, it is useful to conduct a biopsy of the stomach tissue.

The tissue samples taken (a biopsy) from the stomach lining during an endoscopic examination are sent to a lab to be looked at under a microscope. The biopsy is a useful test to see if Helicobacter pylori bacteria are present and to visualize changes in the stomach lining tissue. Other tests may include abdominal x-rays or a barium swallow test that can show the presence of mucosa and thickened folds, which are often signs of inflammation in the stomach.

CHAPTER 2:WHY IS IT DIFFICULT TO CURE GASTRITIS?

Most cases of acute gastritis do not last longer than a few weeks after the patient receives the appropriate treatment from his doctor. However, this does not happen in most cases of chronic gastritis. The problem is that once gastritis appears and becomes chronic, it can be difficult to cure if the possible factors that may be slowing the healing process or making stomach recovery almost impossible are not treated.

Therefore, in this chapter, we will talk about each of the factors that prevent the majority of chronic gastritis cases from being reversed.

It is important that you know that simply not knowing what may be ruining your stomach or preventing it from recovering can make the recovery process much more difficult. Therefore, I recommend that you read this chapter carefully. Having the knowledge or knowing why it is difficult to cure gastritis (especially cases that last a long time) can be very useful when you are creating a treatment plan for gastritis.

What You Eat, Your Habits, and Your Lifestyle

It is possible that at the time your doctor diagnosed you with gastritis, he or she told you what foods you should not eat and those that you can eat as part of the diet to follow to treat gastritis. Apart from that, he or she could have given you some advice and recommendations about the bad habits you should eliminate and the changes you should make in your lifestyle.

However, although this dietary advice and these recommendations are usually useful for starting to treat gastritis, at the same time, they are not accurate or complete regarding all the bad habits you should eliminate, the diet you should follow, and the changes you must make in your lifestyle.

Next, we will talk about the types of foods and beverages, and the most common bad eating habits, that slow down the healing process and prevent inflammation in the stomach from decreasing.

Irritating Foods and Beverages

One of the most common mistakes that people who suffer from gastritis make is eating food and drinking drinks that cause direct and indirect damage to the stomach lining. Foods that can cause direct damage to the stomach lining are mainly all those that are acidic—or, specifically, those that have a pH of less than 4. Foods that do not cause direct damage are those that do so through the stimulation of irritants such as stomach acid and pepsin.

Among the acidic foods we can mention are citrus fruits such as lemons, oranges, tangerines, grapefruit, etc., and acidic fruits such as pineapples, passion fruit, tamarinds, pomegranates, plums, kiwis, green apples, cherries, grapes, and berries (strawberries, blueberries, blackberries, etc.). Among the acidic vegetables we have tomato, tomatillo, and pickles. Most of these foods have a pH of less than 4, which makes them acidic enough to activate pepsin and cause stomach problems.

Some condiments and spices, such as black and white pepper, chili peppers, curry, salt, garlic, and onions, are usually not as acidic as the foods mentioned above but they can irritate the stomach lining when the mucosal barrier that protects it from gastric juices and irritating substances is compromised. However, while such spices and condiments may worsen the symptoms of gastritis, these items by themselves (except for some) do not cause gastritis in a person with a healthy stomach.

In a study conducted in 1987, healthy individuals were given a small dose of black and red peppercorns to see the effect that these spices had on the stomach lining. In that study, it was observed that both black and red peppercorns caused damage to the stomach lining of healthy volunteers.[24] However, in another study, conducted in 1988, about 30 grams of ground jalapeño pepper were placed directly in the stomachs of healthy individuals, to investigate the effect of spicy foods on the stomach lining. After 24 hours the volunteers had an endoscopy; surprisingly, no visible damage was found in the stomach linings of these individuals.[25]

As you can see, the conclusion of the first study was that the consumption of black and red peppercorns can cause irritation in the stomachs of healthy individuals. Meanwhile, the second study concluded that meals prepared with chili pepper are not associated with demonstrable damage to the stomach linings of healthy people. That said, while some spices can irritate the stomach and others can even have gastroprotective effects,[26] the truth is that once inflammation in the stomach is present, spicy foods can worsen gastritis and gastric symptoms associated with this disease, such as stomachache, nausea, and burning sensations, among others.

On the other hand, with respect to acidic or irritating drinks, soft drinks and most store-bought juices and beverages can be mentioned. Those drinks that are usually packaged in cans, plastic, glass bottles, and other beverage containers are subjected to a preservation process in which acidulants (food additives) are added to modify their acidity. Some of the most commonly used acidulants are citric acid, phosphoric acid, lactic acid, ascorbic acid (vitamin C), malic acid, vinegar, and lemon. However, the aforementioned acidic beverages are not the only ones to which said acidulants are added, as many canned or semi-solid foods (jams, baby foods, etc.) found in supermarkets are also acidified. The idea of adding acidulants to these food products is not only to better preserve them but to also improve their flavor and aroma.

If you usually consume such beverages or packaged foods, the next time you go to the supermarket, take a look at the ingredients on the labels of those products. You will see that most of them have been acidified with some of the acidulants mentioned above.

Coffee is another acidic beverage that irritates the stomach lining, both directly and indirectly. Caffeine, which is a stimulating substance found naturally in coffee beans, cocoa, yerba mate, and green and black tea leaves, stimulates acid secretion through the activation of certain bitter taste receptors located in the stomach and oral cavity.[27] On the other hand, the acidity of coffee contributes to the activation of the proteolytic enzyme pepsin, which, together with stomach acid, can cause much more irritation in the stomach, especially if it is empty. In a study conducted in 1981, the effect of decaffeinated coffee was compared to the effect of protein-rich meals on stomach acid secretion. It was discovered that decaffeinated coffee can stimulate gastric acid secretion in a more powerful way than protein-rich meals.[28]

Alcoholic beverages are other types of drinks that we must mention due to the direct damage that ethanol (alcohol) inflicts on the stomach lining. The severity of damage to the stomach lining caused by alcoholic beverages is directly related to the amount of alcohol in the beverage and the frequency with which it is consumed. Beer and wine usually have a pH or acidity level of less than 4, which means that apart from activating pepsin, they cause direct damage to the stomach lining. On the other hand, fermented and non-distilled alcoholic beverages (for example, wine and beer) increase stomach acid secretion. Apparently, succinic acid and other organic acids that contain certain fermented alcoholic beverages are the substances responsible for stimulating gastric acid secretion.[29,30]

Bad Eating Habits

Now that you know about some of the foods and beverages that can directly and indirectly irritate your stomach lining, let's talk about how bad eating habits can worsen gastritis and the symptoms associated with it.

However, before we start, I would like to clarify that, in most cases, the bad eating habits that we will talk about below are not direct causes of gastritis. Rather, they are usually present at the moment it appears. Therefore, taking into account that sometimes gastritis is caused by multiple factors, it is possible that, by themselves, most of these bad habits were not the definitive triggers of your gastritis. Instead, they may have contributed to the appearance of it once they were combined with chronic stress, excessive consumption of alcohol or non-steroidal anti-inflammatory drugs, and other possible triggers.

Now let's review the most common bad habits that might be preventing your stomach from recovering.

Skipping meals. When you spend many hours without eating, your stomach acid and pepsin can wear down the mucus layer and irritate the stomach lining more easily. This happens because when food is in the stomach, it helps absorb irritating substances such as stomach acid and pepsin. When the stomach is empty, its lining is exposed to the corrosive and irritating action of these substances.[31]

Eating too much salt. Salt is a compound that is widely used in world cuisine because of its ability to enhance the flavors of food. However, when it is consumed in excess, it can irritate the stomach lining and cause more inflammation. In a study conducted with people infected with Helicobacter pylori, it was observed that this bacteria is much more aggressive in those who consume a lot of salt in their diets.[32]

Eating hard-to-chew foods. Those who suffer from gastritis usually have stomach discomfort when they eat foods that have a hard consistency or that are difficult to chew. Most of the time, this is because when food is hard to chew, it causes mechanical or frictional irritation in the stomach lining. For example, raw vegetables are usually among the hard foods that cause more problems in those who suffer from gastritis. The fact that a food must be chewed a lot before you can swallow it is a clear indication that it will be difficult to digest and might cause problems in your stomach.

Eating very cold or very hot foods. When it comes to the temperature of food or beverages, keep in mind that very hot or very cold foods and beverages can significantly worsen the irritation and inflammation of the stomach lining.

Eating processed foods. In our society, it is common to see many people who, for lack of time (or simply for pleasure), consume processed and junk food, such as hamburgers, hot dogs, pizza, French fries, biscuits, cakes, candies, cookies, breakfast cereals, instant soups, sausages, etc. However, although for most people this type of processed food is very tempting, what many of them do not realize is that in the long term, the consumption of junk and processed foods can negatively affect one's overall health. Most processed foods contain high levels of bad fats, salt, refined sugars, condiments, and countless additives that irritate the stomach lining and cause inflammation within the body.

On the other hand, there are other bad eating habits that, while they do not directly irritate the stomach lining, can make food digestion much more difficult and, consequently, significantly increase stomach irritation and inflammation. Let's look at those eating habits.

Overeating. One of the main reasons why overeating is bad for you is that when you eat too much, the food stays longer in the stomach. The longer the food stays in the stomach, the greater the likelihood that the stomach lining will be irritated, as it will be exposed to stomach acid and pepsin for longer periods of time. Stomach distension or expansion also causes greater stomach acid release.[33]

Drinking water while eating. Although many people say that drinking water or any other liquid while eating is bad, the truth is that water plays an important role in the digestive process. Some of the chemical reactions in which digestive enzymes participate require water. For that reason, the stomach secretes water along with mucus, stomach acid, and digestive enzymes. However, the problem occurs when you drink large amounts of water while eating, as when you drink a lot of water, you dilute the concentration of stomach acid. This forces your stomach to produce more acid until it reaches an adequate pH level to break down certain foods that require an acidic environment to be digested.

Not chewing food properly. One of the most common habits among people is to chew food a couple of times and then swallow it quickly so that they can eat the next bite. While for some healthy people this may not seem like a problem, those who suffer from digestive problems must eliminate this bad habit. The importance of good chewing is that when you chew food well, a greater surface area will be available so that stomach acid and digestive enzymes can break down food more easily. This, in turn, will make digestion much faster and allow the stomach to work more efficiently.

Eating fatty foods. One of the main reasons why it is not advisable to consume fatty foods when one is suffering from gastritis is that fats decrease gastric emptying and make the stomach lining spend more time in contact with stomach acid and pepsin. As we mentioned earlier, the longer the stomach lining stays in contact with stomach acid, the greater the likelihood of it being irritated. Fats enhance the irritating action of not only stomach acid and pepsin but also of irritating foods and anything that can irritate the stomach lining. Therefore, following a low-fat diet is key for the stomach to recover.

Poor food combining. Another very common bad habit is combining foods improperly—specifically high-protein foods with many carbohydrates or starches. Protein-rich foods require an acidic environment to be broken down, while carbohydrates require an alkaline or neutral environment. Therefore, when protein-rich foods and carbohydrates are eaten together, digestion becomes more complicated, as the enzyme that breaks down carbohydrates is inactivated in a very acidic environment. This, in turn, causes carbohydrates to remain much longer in the stomach, thus increasing the likelihood of the stomach lining becoming irritated and of the appearance of symptoms of acid reflux and indigestion.

A Stressful Life

You might have heard that being in a state of constant stress is not good for your health and that leading a stressful lifestyle can make you sick over time. While all of that is true, what you might not know is that stress and gastritis often go hand in hand.

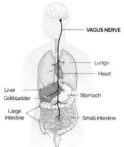

Through research, it has been shown that the brain and the digestive system are closely connected and that they communicate with each other through the vagus nerve, which is one of the most important binding channels in the body. In itself, the digestive system is extremely sensitive to changes in mood and vice versa. In fact, health experts now see stress and anxiety as the main causes of digestive problems such as irritable bowel syndrome, acid reflux, dyspepsia, and, of course, gastritis.[34]

On the other hand, it has long been believed that stress increases the production of stomach acid and, consequently, leads to erosions and ulcers in the stomach lining. And while it is true that the production of too much stomach acid can lead to erosions and ulcers in the stomach, what is really not quite true is that stress causes your stomach to produce excess acid. In fact, one of the reasons why many people perceive or feel that their stomachs produce a lot of acid when they are stressed is that stress decreases the production of gastric mucus, bicarbonate, and other defense mechanisms of the stomach,[10] which, in turn, allows stomach acid, pepsin, and other substances to easily irritate the stomach, making you believe that your stomach is producing excess acid.

Thus, it is important that you know that digestion and all the processes that are carried out in the digestive system are controlled by the enteric nervous system, also known as "the second brain", which is a fully autonomous system that is composed of hundreds of millions of nerve fibers and that communicates with the central nervous system (the brain) through the vagus nerve. When you are stressed, a response is activated in your body known as "fight or flight," which decreases gastric secretions (including the production of gastric mucus and bicarbonate), interferes with muscle contractions along the gastrointestinal tract, and restricts blood to the gastrointestinal mucosa and the entire digestive system. All this happens so that you can use your body's resources to face the stressful situation.

Stress and a hectic lifestyle can not only negatively affect your digestive system but also lead you to develop unhealthy habits, including many of the bad habits we mentioned earlier. For example, alcohol consumption is a very common habit among those who lead stressful lives. Many of them see this bad habit as a way to relax or escape everything that causes them stress; however, what many people do not know is that alcohol consumption is one of the unhealthy habits that can most affect the stomach, as alcohol is a toxic substance that is highly irritating to the stomach lining.

Smoking is another bad habit that many people use as a way to deal with stress. However, the nicotine in cigarettes increases stomach acid and pepsin secretion and, at the same time, significantly decreases the stomach's defenses,[8] thus favoring the appearance of gastritis and ulcers in the stomach lining.

Finally, it is important to clarify that when we talk about stress, we refer not only to stress at work or daily stress; in fact, emotional stress (including anxiety and depression) can affect your stomach just as much as, or even more severely than, any other type of stress. Some studies have found that psychological or emotional stress and depression are related to various digestive diseases and may be risk factors for functional dyspepsia, irritable bowel syndrome, and peptic ulcers.[34]

The Damage of Stomach Acid and Pepsin

In terms of why it is difficult to cure gastritis, especially chronic and more severe cases, you should know that healing the stomach is not like healing a wound in the arm. Unlike an external wound, the stomach lining is constantly attacked by stomach acid and pepsin, which create an environment that is not conducive for the stomach lining to recover.

Therefore, to create a therapeutic strategy or treatment plan that allows you to effectively reduce inflammation in the stomach, you must first know the aggressive factors that can most affect the stomach lining. This way, you will know what to do and how to minimize the damage that these aggressive factors can inflict on your stomach lining.

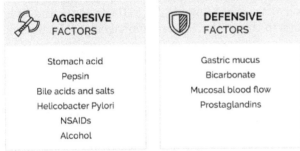

In the previous image, we could see the most common aggressive factors of the stomach lining, as well as the main defense mechanisms of the same. Stomach acid and pepsin represent the aggressive factors of the stomach lining and are the main products of gastric secretion capable of inducing mucosal injury. Mucus and bicarbonate are two of the main components of the so-called mucosal barrier that protects the stomach lining.

Gastric mucus is divided into two layers: the inner layer and the outer layer. The inner layer, also called adherent mucus, forms a gelatinous coating with a high concentration of bicarbonate that helps maintain a neutral pH (7.0), thus protecting the stomach lining from stomach acid. The main function of bicarbonate is to significantly weaken the acidity of gastric juices to prevent secreted acid from returning to the cell and damaging the stomach lining. On the other hand, the outer layer, or soluble mucus, is a less viscous layer that mixes with food and harmful agents in the stomach, then detaches itself from the inner layer. Both layers are part of the physicochemical barrier that separates the stomach lining from the gastric lumen. The protection offered by the mucosal barrier is the reason why the stomach cannot self-digest itself.[35]

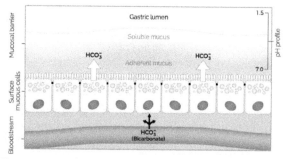

Damage to the stomach lining mucosa occurs when there is an imbalance between aggressive factors and protective factors. A combination of aggressive factors that can lead to the appearance of gastritis and gastric ulcers is an excessive intake of alcohol, being under a state of constant stress, and consuming non-steroidal anti-inflammatory drugs. The combination of these three factors results in a decrease in the pH gradient through the mucus-bicarbonate barrier and in greater exposure of the lining to stomach acid and pepsin.

Stomach Acid

Stomach acid, also known as hydrochloric acid, is a highly corrosive substance secreted by parietal cells. The main function of this substance is to: break down food into molecules that are easily degraded in their passage through the gastrointestinal tract; convert pepsinogen into its active form, which is pepsin; and give the stomach a fairly low pH range (between 1 and 2) to allow pepsin to initiate protein digestion and to allow the lower esophageal sphincter and pylorus to be properly stimulated.

Stomach acid is also the first line of defense against bacteria and pathogens that try to enter the body through food. Therefore, its presence and low levels of gastric acidity favor the elimination of bacteria and pathogens.

One of the most important things you should know about stomach acid is what really causes its release in the stomach. Knowing this is really useful, as with that information you can create a plan that allows you to minimize the release of this substance and the damage that it can inflict on your stomach lining.

The secretion of stomach acid and other substances necessary for digestion is carried out in three phases.[36] The amount of acid that the stomach secretes can vary in each of the following phases:

1.   **Cephalic phase:** When you smell, think, taste, or see food, your stomach receives signals from the upper centers of the brain (through the vagus nerve via the neurotransmitter acetylcholine) that cause it to release stomach acid, pepsinogen, and gastric mucus. In this phase, approximately thirty percent of the total stomach acid is secreted before food enters the stomach.[37]

2.   **Gastric phase:** About sixty percent of total stomach acid is secreted in this phase. The gastric phase of acid secretion begins when food comes into contact with the stomach lining. Ingested food stimulates gastric acid secretion through the distension or expansion of the stomach (by short and long reflexes via acetylcholine) and the presence of proteins (small peptides and amino acids) in the food. The interaction of food proteins with stomach G cells causes them to release a hormone called gastrin into the bloodstream. This hormone, which directly stimulates parietal cells, is considered the most potent stimulant of gastric acid secretion. Therefore, the more protein-rich foods you eat, the greater the release response of that hormone.[36]

3.   **Intestinal phase:** In this last phase, the gastric acid secretion decreases dramatically once partially digested food reaches the small intestine. About five to ten percent of total stomach acid secretion is secreted at this stage. Apparently, the distension of the wall of the small intestine (specifically of the duodenum) and the presence of amino acids and peptides are responsible for slightly stimulating gastric acid secretion. However, once the small intestine detects fats and low acidity levels (or a pH less than 3), it releases inhibitory hormones to stop the gastric acid secretion.[36]

There is also another phase of gastric acid secretion known as the interdigestive phase. In this phase, there is a small continuous basal acid secretion between meals and while you sleep. A circadian rhythm is observed in which the basal acid secretion reaches its maximum levels while you sleep and its lowest point during the first hours of the morning.[36] Scientific evidence shows that this nocturnal acid secretion depends largely on a stimulus on the parietal cells caused by histamine, which is a substance that acts as a hormone and neurotransmitter in the body.[38]

On the other hand, one of the phases of gastric acid secretion to which you should pay more attention is the gastric phase, as it is the phase during which the greatest amount of stomach acid is secreted and over which you can have greater control. One of the things that you can do is to control the amount of food you eat to avoid a greater distention of the stomach, which will cause the stomach to secrete less acid.

Although this could help significantly, the greatest benefit could be obtained by avoiding certain foods and drinks that greatly stimulate gastric acid secretion. The drinks that most stimulate gastric acid secretion are coffee, milk, beer, and wine.[39] The foods that most stimulate gastric acid secretion are all those that are rich in protein—mainly those of animal origin (including milk and eggs).

However, unlike the drinks mentioned above, you cannot stop consuming proteins, as they play an important role in the repair and regeneration of damaged tissues. Therefore, in the next chapter, we will talk about some strategies that you can implement to continue supplying your body with the proteins and amino acids it needs to repair damaged tissues.

Another thing that is not advisable to do when you are suffering from gastritis is to chew gum on an empty stomach. When you chew gum, the cephalic phase of acid secretion is activated,[40] which deceives the stomach, making it think that food is on its way. The problem with this is that once the acid is released in your stomach and there is no food to be digested, the stomach acid will start to irritate and inflame your stomach lining. In addition, chewing gums are not very good for your health, as most contain artificial flavorings, refined sugar, preservatives, and other ingredients that can further irritate your stomach.

Now that you know how stomach acid is secreted, what its function is in the stomach, and the damage that it can cause to the stomach lining, let's talk about pepsin and how this substance can cause even more damage in the stomach.

Pepsin

The first thing you should know is that pepsin is nothing more than a digestive enzyme produced by the chief cells. When you eat food, your stomach releases pepsin in its inactive form (known as pepsinogen), which requires an acidic environment to be converted into pepsin. Pepsin's function is to partially break down food proteins (for example, meat and eggs) into peptides, which then pass into the small intestine, where other proteolytic enzymes break down the peptides into amino acids, which are then absorbed and used by the body.[41]

The conversion of pepsinogen into pepsin is slow at a pH of 6 but extremely fast at a pH of 2 or lower. However, once pepsin is activated, for it to function, it needs an environment with a pH of less than 5 because its enzymatic activity is virtually non-existent in less acidic environments. The ideal environment for this enzyme to act, or for the proper breakdown of food proteins, is a pH of between 1.5 and 2.5.[42]

The problem with pepsin is that it is activated not only by stomach acid but also by any food or beverage that acidifies the stomach content or that has a pH lower than 5. Examples include citrus or acidic fruits, tomatoes, pickles, vinegar, salad dressings, ketchup, fermented beverages (including beer and wine), soft drinks, and most store-bought beverages that have been acidified with acidulants. Each time you consume acidic foods or drinks, such as those mentioned above, you contribute to the activation of pepsin, which, in turn, leads to increased wear of the mucosal barrier and, consequently, to more inflammation and irritation in your stomach.

On the other hand, pepsin can irritate not only your stomach lining but also the lining of your esophagus. When you experience acid reflux, the pepsin rises to the esophagus and inflames the tissues of the esophagus, which, unlike the stomach, does not have a mucosal barrier that protects it from the corrosive action of stomach acid and pepsin. Once this enzyme rises to the esophagus, it is planted and sits in it. It remains inactive (because the pH inside the esophagus is usually higher than 6) until it is reactivated by subsequent events of acid reflux or by some food or acidic drink.

This enzyme is inactivated in an environment with a pH greater than 6.5 but remains stable until pH 7.5, so it can be reactivated by coming into contact with an acidic environment (for example, acidic foods or drinks). However, once pepsin is exposed to an environment with a pH greater than 7.5, it is completely denatured and irreversibly inactivated.[42]

In the next chapter, you will find a list of foods that have a pH higher than 5 and of all those irritating foods that you should eliminate from your diet. Apart from this, you will find a list of tips and recommendations regarding all the bad habits you should eliminate and the changes you should make in your lifestyle to heal your stomach.

CHAPTER 3: THE HEALING PROGRAM

Now that you know what gastritis is and why it is difficult to cure, we will start with the healing program. In this healing program, you must establish a base healing during the first 90 days. From there, the healing process of your stomach will be easier and you can recover faster from any flare-ups that you may have.

The main objective of this healing program is to attack gastritis from all angles simultaneously. That is why it focuses on three main parts: diet, habits, and stress/mental health. By attacking gastritis from these three angles, you will more quickly reduce the inflammation and damage that stomach acid and pepsin have inflicted on your stomach lining.

It is important to clarify that the 90-day period is subjective, as some people can recover in less time (this depends on the type of gastritis you suffer from and its severity). However, experience has taught me that it takes at least 90 days to establish a solid base healing.

The first critical step you should take to reduce inflammation and irritation in your stomach is to eliminate from your diet all foods that can irritate your stomach lining and prevent it from recovering. The diet for gastritis should not only eliminate foods that irritate or cause inflammation in the stomach but also include foods that nourish your body, help fight inflammation, and regenerate the stomach lining. Therefore, I recommend that, during the first 90 days, you not limit your diet beyond avoiding those foods that are not recommended for consumption (with the exception of allowed foods that you do not tolerate). Doing this is intended to reduce the likelihood that you will suffer from malnutrition in the future.

Following this, we will move on to the second step, in which we will talk about all the bad habits that you should eliminate to avoid worsening your stomach or exacerbating symptoms related to gastritis. This step includes making some changes to your lifestyle.

After we talk about all the bad habits that you should eliminate and the changes you must make in your lifestyle, we will move on to the third step, in which we will talk about stress and anxiety and how both negatively affect the stomach and your overall health. This third step is extremely important, as stress and anxiety are among the main triggers of gastritis. Therefore, if you don't learn how to manage them, it will be much harder for your stomach to recover.

Finally, to strengthen the healing program, the fourth chapter and the third part of the book have been included. In the fourth chapter, you will find a list of remedies and supplements that will help you repair and regenerate your stomach lining faster. In the third part of the book, you will find a one-week meal plan and more than 50 gastritis-friendly and gluten- and dairy-free recipes. Both the meal plan and the recipes were included to make it easier for you to follow the gastritis diet that we will talk about next.

FIRST STEP

Change Your Diet

In this first step, you will eliminate from your diet all the foods and beverages that can irritate your stomach lining and, then, introduce into your diet foods that help fight inflammation and facilitate the recovery of your stomach. Doing this is essential and very important, as you might never get better if you do not get rid of everything that may be irritating your stomach and causing more inflammation in it.

First, we will talk about all the foods that you should avoid eating. Then we will talk about the five types of foods that you should include in your diet.

• **Acidic fruits.** Avoid eating citrus fruits such as lemons, oranges, tangerines, grapefruit, etc., and acidic fruits such as pineapples, passion fruit, tamarinds, pomegranates, plums, kiwis, green apples, cherries, grapes, and berries (strawberries, blueberries, blackberries, etc.). All these fruits have a pH lower than 4, which makes them acidic enough to activate pepsin and further irritate the stomach lining. (Later, I will give you some tips on how to safely consume some of these acidic fruits.) On the other hand, it is important to clarify that one of the reasons why some people can tolerate lemon is because of the type of gastritis from which they suffer. People who suffer from superficial non-erosive gastritis with low production of stomach acid, tend to tolerate lemon well. Those with erosive and more severe gastritis usually have more problems when they consume lemon or something that contains it.

• **Vegetables and irritating condiments.** Some of the vegetables you should avoid are onion, garlic, bell pepper, tomato, tomatillo, and pickles. Among the spices and condiments that you should avoid are chili peppers, black and white peppercorns, curry, mint, ketchup, mustard, mayonnaise, barbecue or tomato sauce, vinegar, hot sauces, and salad dressings. Spicy meals should also be avoided.

• **Sugary and soft drinks.** Most store-bought juices and beverages that come in bottles, cans, and other containers should be avoided because they contain added citric acid and/or other acidulants. Carbonation is also bad for gastritis, so it is better to avoid any carbonated beverage, including sparkling water.

• **Caffeinated drinks.** Avoid drinking beverages that contain caffeine, such as coffee, hot chocolate, energy drinks, and most herbal teas. Caffeine relaxes the lower esophageal sphincter and stimulates gastric acid secretion.[43] You can substitute most herbal teas and strong teas (such as green or black tea) with others that do not contain caffeine. Some of the herbal teas that do not have caffeine (and that are safe to consume) are chamomile, licorice, marshmallow root, fennel, ginger, lavender, and anise teas. Coffee can be substituted with chicory root, also known as chicory coffee, which is an excellent caffeine-free substitute with a taste very similar to coffee.

• **Alcoholic drinks.** Any type of beverage that is classified as "alcoholic" can irritate your stomach lining. Therefore, I recommend that you avoid consuming any beverage that contains alcohol. Beer and wine, apart from containing alcohol, are also acidic and stimulate gastric acid secretion.[44]

• **Processed foods.** You should avoid processed and junk food, as these do not provide a true nutritional benefit to the body. All they do is slow down the healing process and increase intestinal inflammation. Some of the foods to avoid are cookies, biscuits, cakes, candies, donuts, chocolate, breakfast cereals, white bread, pasta, popcorn, French fries, pizza, processed meats, sausages, and instant soups. Most processed foods and canned foods (or packaged foods) are loaded with food additives, dyes, refined sugars, and artificial sweeteners that negatively affect your health. Therefore, just as a poor diet is, in most cases, part of the problem, whole and healthy food consumption must be part of the solution.

• **Fatty foods.** One of the most important things you should do in your diet is avoid fatty foods and all types of fried foods, since, as we mentioned earlier, fats decrease gastric emptying and slow the digestion of other foods. Fast food and baked goods contain many trans fats—a type of unhealthy fat that, when consumed in excess, can be harmful to the body. It is recommended that you also avoid refined vegetable oils such as soybean oil, corn oil, canola oil, and sunflower oil as much as possible, as the production of these seed oils requires an industrial process that involves the use of very high temperatures (which destabilizes the molecular structure of these oils) and of chemicals such as hexane solvent. Instead of frying your food, you can sauté it with a little coconut, olive, or avocado oil.

• **Dairy products.** It is recommended that you avoid the consumption of cow's milk and dairy products. The proteins contained in cow's milk stimulate gastric acid secretion, while its saturated fat decreases gastric emptying. This combination of many fats and proteins can further irritate the stomach lining. The main protein component of cow's milk is beta-casein. The most frequent variants are beta-casein A1 and A2. Recent studies have shown that cow's milk that contains beta-casein A1 (the most common in supermarkets) promotes intestinal inflammation and exacerbates gastrointestinal symptoms.[45] Some products and foods that also contain dairy are cheeses, ice cream, yogurt, custard, butter, whey protein, condensed milk, and milk-based desserts.

• **Gluten.** You may not have any problem eating foods with gluten, which is a glycoprotein found mainly in cereals such as wheat, rye, and barley. However, gluten is difficult to digest and alters intestinal permeability (i.e., damages the walls of the intestine).[46] When the intestine becomes more permeable, more toxins pass into your bloodstream, which increases inflammation at the intestinal level and causes an elevated immune response. Therefore, I recommend that you avoid eating any food that contains gluten during the first two or three months while trying to reduce inflammation in your stomach. Some foods that contain gluten are white and whole wheat bread, breakfast cereals, pasta, muffins, pizza, cookies, cakes, and any food made with wheat flour.

By eliminating from your diet all the foods we have mentioned above, you will not only facilitate the recovery of your stomach lining but also help reduce inflammation both in the intestines and throughout your body. Now we will talk about the five types of foods you should consume and include in your diet.

#1: Foods with a pH Higher Than 5

For at least the first 90 days, you must consume only foods that have a pH level higher than 5. This will help suppress the activity of pepsin, which is necessary for the inflammation and irritation in the stomach to decrease faster.

The following is not a definitive or complete list, but here are some foods that have a pH greater than 5:

• **Fruits:** papaya, melon, watermelon, banana, dragon fruit, avocado, and black olives. Among pears, the less acidic varieties (which it is recommended that you eat) are Bosc and Asian. Always try to consume fruits when they are ripe, never unripe.

• **Vegetables:** spinach, kale, broccoli, cauliflower, arugula, celery, Brussels sprouts, chard, artichoke, asparagus, zucchini, okra, mushrooms, carrots, beets, chayote, pumpkin and squash (all varieties), parsnips, jicama, turnip, yam, potatoes, sweet potato, and malanga (taro). Most vegetables have a pH higher than 5, so don't worry too much.

• **Herbs and condiments:** coriander, rosemary, parsley, sage, thyme, basil, oregano, coriander, saffron, asafetida, sumac, bay leaves, dill, tarragon, star anise, celery seeds, cumin seeds, fennel seeds, coriander seeds, sea salt or Himalayan salt, Bragg liquid aminos or coconut aminos (alternatives to soy sauce), extra virgin olive oil, coconut oil, avocado oil, and hemp oil. Always choose cold-pressed vegetable oils, as they are of higher quality, better preserve their nutritional values, and have not been refined or chemically extracted.

• **Poultry:** skinless chicken or turkey breast and eggs. Chicken or turkey legs and thighs are known as dark meat, which has a higher fat content. If available, choose organic chicken or turkey breasts, and organic eggs. I also recommend that you avoid eating red meat, as it contains large amounts of saturated fat and is much harder to digest.

- **Fish and seafood:** tilapia, trout, herring, wild salmon, cod, sardines, anchovies, small mackerel, flounder, haddock, hake, catfish, sole, lobster, scallop, crab, and shrimp. It is advisable that you eat as little as possible of fish such as swordfish, grouper, marlin, king or Spanish mackerel, and albacore, as they contain high levels of mercury. Mercury is a dangerous and highly toxic heavy metal for the human body. When it accumulates in the body, mercury can adversely affect the nervous and immune systems.[47] The larger and older the fish, the more mercury it can contain.

- **Others:** almond milk, rice milk, or other plant-based milks (as alternatives to cow's milk), coconut water, alkaline water, pure maple syrup, stevia, monk fruit, vanilla extract, and almond butter. Peanut butter is allowed so long as it is organic and does not contain hydrogenated oils.

This list does not include foods such as beans, legumes (soybeans, peas, chickpeas, lentils, etc.), whole grains (corn, rye, barley, wheat, sorghum, spelt, brown rice, etc.), and nightshades (tomato, peppers, and eggplants) because they are usually more difficult to digest and can cause intestinal symptoms such as bloating, gas, and stomach cramps, among others. In addition, these foods contain high levels of antinutrients such as phytates (phytic acid), lectins, and enzyme inhibitors, which are substances that reduce the absorption of nutrients in the small intestine and significantly decrease the nutritional value of these foods.[48]

Although antinutrients are not a major concern for most people, they can become a problem during periods of malnutrition or poor nutrient absorption. Therefore, it is recommended that you replace whole grains with tubers such as potato, sweet potato, malanga (taro), cassava, yam, etc. White rice is easier to digest and does not contain as many antinutrients as brown rice, so it is one of the few grains (along with instant unflavored or quick-cooking oats) that you can consume at the beginning.

Nuts and seeds were also not included in this list, as they contain high levels of antinutrients and have a high fat content, which makes them much more difficult to digest. However, most of the mentioned foods (nuts, seeds, legumes, beans, and whole grains) can be reintroduced into the diet after the first 90 days have passed. It is recommended that before you consume them, they be "activated" to reduce the amount of antinutrients, make them more digestible, and ensure that your body can more easily obtain the nutrients that these foods contain.

There are many methods to "activate" or reduce the antinutrient levels of such foods. Some of these methods are soaking, germination, fermentation, and boiling. However, the most effective way to reduce antinutrients in food is to combine different elimination methods. Through a combination of different methods, many antinutrients can degrade almost completely. For example, one study found that soaking, germinating, and fermenting decrease phytic acid in quinoa by 98 percent.[49] Similar results were found with corn and sorghum by combining several methods to reduce their levels of antinutrients.[50]

On the other hand, bananas help coat the stomach lining and, being rich in potassium, act as a natural antacid. However, some people who suffer from gastritis often experience acid reflux, heartburn, and stomach upset when they consume bananas. My recommendation is that you always try to consume bananas when they are very ripe (preferably when they have brown spots on the skin), as in this way they are usually more gastritis-friendly.

Cruciferous vegetables such as broccoli, cauliflower, Brussels sprouts, and cabbage also often cause intestinal discomfort in some people (especially those suffering from irritable bowel syndrome). Therefore, you should keep in mind that not everyone is equal and that, depending on the type of gastritis from which you suffer, your stomach will react differently to certain foods.

My recommendation is to see for yourself whether you tolerate some of these mentioned foods. The idea here is to initially avoid all foods that are difficult to digest or that can cause stomach discomfort.

#2: Antioxidant-Rich Foods

It is important that you maintain a high consumption of antioxidants and flavonoid-rich foods, as these will not only help reduce inflammation in the stomach but also accelerate the repair of gastric tissue that has been damaged by stomach acid, pepsin, and other irritating substances.[51]

The main function of antioxidants is to eliminate free radicals and protect cells from the damage that free radicals cause when they are produced excessively.[52] Meanwhile, flavonoids—substances found in fruits and vegetables—have been shown to possess strong anti-inflammatory and antioxidant properties.[53] Therefore, eating foods rich in both antioxidants and flavonoids can be very beneficial in treating gastritis.

Flavonoid-rich vegetables that also contain considerable amounts of antioxidant vitamins such as A and C include spinach, kale, broccoli, Brussels sprouts, chard, arugula, celery, okra, artichokes, asparagus, and green leafy vegetables. It is recommended that you consume at least one pound of this type of vegetable daily, preferably steamed, roasted, or lightly sautéed in a pan. Unlike other cooking methods, those mentioned above offer a lower loss of antioxidants and nutrients in most vegetables.[54] However, no cooking method is perfect when it comes to retaining antioxidants or nutrients in vegetables, as not all vegetables behave in the same way when exposed to the same cooking methods.[55] It should also be taken into account that the time that a portion of food is exposed to heat can affect its final antioxidant and nutrient content. The longer a food is cooked, the greater the loss of nutrients. Therefore, to retain as many antioxidants and nutrients as possible during cooking, cook your vegetables for only half the typical time. This means you will enjoy your vegetables a little crunchier (as long as you can tolerate them that way).

Other foods that can be mentioned, mostly because of their beta-carotene and other antioxidant content, are carrots, beets, squash, and sweet potatoes.

On the other hand, most fruits that are rich in antioxidants and flavonoids, usually have a pH less than 5. Eating those fruits may not be very good for a stomach that is irritated and inflamed. However, my recommendation is that you avoid consuming most acidic fruits on an empty stomach; try to mix them with alkaline foods to help neutralize their acidity. (We'll talk about this shortly.)

Among the acidic fruits that have a pH of less than 5 are blueberries, strawberries, blackberries, raspberries, cherries, peaches, apricots, kiwi, mango, plums, grapes, pears (except Bosc and Asian varieties), and green apples. (The least acidic apple is the Red Delicious variety.) A safe way to consume these fruits is to mix them with alkaline foods to neutralize their acidity. Smoothies made with almond milk are an excellent way to consume most of these acidic fruits and take advantage of their nutrients while preventing pepsin from activating.

When preparing your smoothies, you can use one part of these acidic fruits for every two parts of almond milk or any other plant-based milk you use (taking into account that some plant-based milks may be less alkaline than others). For example, for every cup of strawberries you use in your smoothies, you will add two cups of almond milk. In this way, you make sure that the final pH of the smoothie is not as acidic, as you will neutralize the acidity of the fruit.

Finally, it is recommended that you consume at least one or two cups of fruit daily. Just keep in mind that it is preferable that you consume in your smoothies those fruits that have a pH of less than 5, while those that have a pH of greater than 5 (such as papaya, bananas, melon, watermelon, etc.) can be consumed both in smoothies and on an empty stomach. Also, try to ensure that much of your fruit consumption comes from those fruits that are rich in vitamins C and A and flavonoids. Such fruits include papaya, cantaloupe melon, strawberries, blueberries, raspberries, among others.

#3: Essential Fatty Acid-Rich Foods

Fats play an important role in the body, as they help absorb fat-soluble vitamins such as A, D, E, and K, which must be transported by fat molecules through the bloodstream. In addition, fats are used as energy sources by the body and have an essential function in the formation of hormones.

In general, fats are classified into good fats (polyunsaturated and monounsaturated) and bad fats (trans and saturated). On the other hand, essential fatty acids (EFAs) are a type of good (polyunsaturated) fat that our body cannot synthesize by itself. Therefore, we must obtain it through our diet.

The two main essential fatty acids are linoleic acid (omega-6) and alpha-linolenic acid (omega-3). Omega-3 fatty acids help reduce inflammation in the body and are necessary for the proper functioning of the brain and nervous system.[56] Meanwhile, omega-6 fatty acids perform important functions in the body in relation to cardiovascular and hormonal health and to glucose metabolism.

Following are some of the foods that are good sources of essential fatty acids and healthy fats:

• **Fish:** sardines, wild salmon, herring, and small mackerel. These fish are all rich in omega-3 fatty acids.

• **Healthy oils:** extra virgin olive oil, flaxseed oil, walnut oil, avocado oil, and hemp oil. Among these healthy oils, krill oil supplement stands out, as, apart from being one of the best sources of omega-3, it is rich in astaxanthin, a carotenoid with potent antioxidant and anti-inflammatory activity.[57]

• **Seeds and nuts:** cashews, almonds, hazelnuts, walnuts, pecans, pistachios, Brazil nuts, chia seeds, linseed seeds, sunflower seeds, pumpkin seeds, hemp seeds, and sesame seeds.

It is recommended that you reintroduce the nuts and seeds into your diet after the first 90 days, since, as we mentioned earlier, these are more difficult to digest because of their high fat and antinutrient content. Walnuts and shelled hemp seeds are the only exceptions that you can introduce into your diet from the beginning, though only moderately. Of all nuts, walnuts have the highest amount of omega-3 and antioxidant polyphenols,[58] which delivers a double whammy against chronic inflammation. Meanwhile, hemp seeds stand out for being rich in essential fatty acids (omega-3 and omega-6), high-quality proteins, and a variety of minerals.

Thus, it is recommended that you moderately consume the foods rich in omega-3 that we mentioned earlier (for example, salmon, because it has a lot of fat). Remember that because a food is rich in good or healthy fats does not mean that your stomach will tolerate it. Fats (good or bad) delay digestion; the longer digestion lasts, the more the stomach lining will be exposed to stomach acid and pepsin, thus increasing the risk of stomach irritation.

Therefore, when adding healthy fats to your diet, you should introduce them in small amounts. For example, if you want to use olive oil in your favorite salads or dishes, you can start by adding a teaspoon. As you get better, you can increase the amount little by little, without overdoing it with the amount of oil you add to your meals. Avocado is also another food rich in monounsaturated fats that you can moderately include in your diet.

While it is true that omega-3 essential fatty acids can help reduce inflammation in the stomach, it is also important that you maintain a balance between the amount of omega-3 and omega-6 you consume in your diet. Both types of fatty acids are necessary for the body to function properly. Therefore, it is important that you incorporate them into your diet in the right ratios. Official recommendations indicate that the optimal ratio between omega-3 and omega-6 is 1:4 or less.[59]

Some research has shown that linoleic acid, an essential fatty acid of the omega-6 series mentioned earlier, increases the gastric expression of prostaglandin E2, which stimulates the production of gastric mucus, bicarbonate, and other defense mechanisms of the stomach.[60,61] Some linoleic-acid-rich foods are walnuts, sunflower seeds, and hemp seeds.

However, it is important to note that in the synthesis of prostaglandins, the conversion from linoleic acid (LA) to gamma-linoleic acid (GLA), an intermediate of fatty acid biosynthesis, is very slow and is restricted by stress, smoking, alcohol, NSAIDs, excess consumption of saturated and trans fats, and deficiencies of vitamin C, B6, zinc, and magnesium. All these factors affect the activity of the enzyme delta-6-desaturase, which converts linoleic acid into GLA. In terms of avoiding this often inefficient and limiting step in the metabolism of LA to GLA, gamma-linolenic acid supplementation is a better option to ensure adequate synthesis of prostaglandins.[62] Vegetable oils such as evening primrose oil, blackcurrant seed oil, borage seed oil, and hemp seed oil are excellent dietary sources of GLA.

#4: High-Quality, Protein-Rich Foods

Protein is essential to repairing damaged tissues in the stomach and throughout the body. Therefore, it is necessary that you maintain an adequate and moderate intake of protein-rich foods. Fish, chicken, and eggs are good sources of animal protein. These foods provide a good amount of glutamine, an amino acid that not only improves tissue healing but also repairs and keeps the gastrointestinal walls in good condition.

The reason I recommend that protein consumption be moderate is that, as I have already mentioned, foods that are high in protein (mainly those of animal origin) greatly stimulate gastric acid secretion. The more protein you consume in a meal, the more acid and pepsin your stomach will release, which, in turn, can greatly increase inflammation and irritation in stomach lining.

If you have a very sensitive stomach, it would be good to avoid consuming animal protein for at least the first two to four weeks and then moderately reintroduce (in small quantities) chicken or turkey breast, fish, and eggs. By doing this, you will be helping your stomach lining begin to regenerate and causing inflammation to decrease faster.

However, it is not recommended that you stop consuming animal protein without first knowing or planning what you are going to replace it with. Preferably, consult with a nutritionist before doing this. Two good substitutes for animal protein are hemp protein and pea protein powder. These are two sources of plant-based proteins that are easy to digest and that cause your stomach to release less stomach acid.

On the one hand, hemp protein, which is derived from hemp seeds, is considered a good source of plant-based protein because it contains the nine essential amino acids that the body does not produce. It also contains a good variety of vitamins and minerals, such as Vitamin E, B vitamins, magnesium, phosphorus, calcium, iron, potassium, manganese, and zinc. Apart from this, hemp protein is rich in essential fatty acids (omega-6 and omega-3) and is one of the few plant-based sources of gamma-linolenic acid (GLA), which is an essential fatty acid that we talked about earlier and that has also been shown to have anti-inflammatory properties.[63] One of the main components of hemp protein is edestine, which is a highly digestible globular protein that is easily metabolized due to its optimum amino acid composition.[64] Globular proteins are soluble in water, so they dissolve easily and are more easily absorbed by the digestive system.

On the other hand, pea protein, which contains a high content of quality amino acids and proteins, is obtained by extracting soluble protein from split yellow peas. In the extraction process, water and a mechanical process are used to eliminate most of the starch and fiber content, leaving mainly the isolated protein, with some vitamins and minerals. Peas, like other legumes, naturally contain antinutrients that interfere with the absorption of other nutrients, such as proteins, vitamins, and minerals. However, these substances are almost completely eliminated in the extraction process used to create the pea protein isolate.

The only problem with hemp protein and pea protein powder supplements is that they don't provide all the essential amino acids in the amounts that the body needs. So, if you decide to not consume animal protein for a long time, the best thing you can do is combine plant-based proteins to create a protein powder with a complete amino acid profile. A combination that is being widely used by vegans and vegetarians is that of pea protein with rice protein in a 50/50 ratio. Unlike rice protein, pea protein is high in the amino acid lysine but low in other essential amino acids that rice protein contains. When both proteins are combined, they offer an amino acid profile that is comparable to that of whey protein.[65] In fact, in a study conducted in 2015 by the Journal of the International Society for Sports Nutrition, it was found that pea protein can increase muscle thickness as potently as milk proteins, and that it can be used as an alternative to whey-based proteins.[66]

In addition, hemp protein is a less-complete source of protein than peas and contains fewer grams of protein per serving than the latter. Therefore, hemp protein is considered a protein of inferior quality. When one is considering the quality of proteins, it is also important to observe their digestibility. This can be determined using the Protein Digestibility Corrected Amino Acid Score (PDCAAS). A protein that scores 100 percent provides all the essential amino acids. Pea protein has a PDCAAS of 89 percent,[67] while hemp protein has a PDCAAS that averages around 50 percent.[68] This means that pea protein is a better source of essential amino acids than hemp protein and, therefore, is considered a more complete source of plant-based protein.

My final advice is not to stress yourself by wanting to combine rice protein with pea protein unless your protein sources are very limited or if you are eating only very small amounts of food.

Another thing to keep in mind is that when choosing a hemp protein powder supplement, you should try to choose the one with the least amount of fiber per serving. In this way, you will avoid causing problems in your stomach. An excellent way to consume hemp and pea protein is to add it to your smoothies.

#5: Easy-to-Digest Foods

The gastritis diet should always consist of foods that are easy to chew and digest. Therefore, it is necessary that you consume only foods that are soft in consistency and that are not raw. By doing this, you will speed up the recovery of your stomach, as the main objective of eating a bland diet is to facilitate digestion and ensure that the digestive system works as little as possible so that it can recover.

Vegetables and fruits are on the list of easily digested foods. However, fruits should be consumed only when they are ripe. You should avoid consuming on an empty stomach those fruits that have a pH of less than 5. It is preferable that you consume acidic fruits in smoothies made with almond milk. Meanwhile, those with a pH greater than 5 can be consumed both in smoothies and on an empty stomach.

On the other hand, vegetables should never be eaten raw. It is recommended that during the first weeks, you avoid vegetables that are very hard or fibrous. When a food is difficult to chew, it will also be difficult to digest. Therefore, if the digestive system is not working properly, foods that are too hard or fiber-rich may be a burden on it. Fruits with skin, whole grains, legumes, and beans are some of the foods that contain the most fiber.

Cooked foods are softer and easier to digest, so I recommend that you always prepare them steamed, baked, grilled, or sautéed. To give you an idea, following are some cooked foods that are easy to digest and that you can include in your diet at the beginning:

- Purée of potatoes, sweet potatoes, taro, or pumpkin
- Cream of rice
- Almond milk smoothies
- Steamed vegetables
- Homemade chicken or vegetable soup
- Bone broth

Proteins of animal origin, such as chicken or turkey breast and fish, should be consumed without skin and always prepared on the grill, baked, or steamed. Fatty fish such as salmon, sardine, trout, etc., should be consumed in moderation due to its high fat content. If you don't tolerate eggs, start by consuming only the egg whites. As you get better, you can introduce the egg yolk to make preparations such as tortillas and poached, soft-boiled, and hard-boiled eggs.

Tips for Eating Healthy When Eating Out

Eating out is a big challenge for most people who suffer from gastritis, as it is difficult to find restaurants or places that prepare gastritis-friendly meals. However, this does not have to sabotage your efforts to follow a healthy diet that does not worsen your symptoms or stomach problems. Use the following tips to make healthy choices the next time you eat out.

- If you are going to eat in a restaurant, read the menu well and ask the waiter or chef to make small adjustments to the dishes you choose. For example, if a dish you would like to order contains tomato, onion, lemon, hot sauce, or other irritating ingredients, ask the waiter or chef to prepare your dish without that or those particular ingredient(s).

- Always try to choose chicken, turkey, or fish prepared on the grill, baked or steamed, and seasoned only with salt and non-irritating condiments. Vegetables should always be steamed, sauteed, or grilled, without vinegar, lemon, or other irritating dressings. Avoid fried, sauced, or breaded foods and sauces or stews made with unknown ingredients.

- With regard to drinks, whether you are in a restaurant or any other place, it is recommended that you opt for smoothies or fruit juices that you tolerate (as long as they are available). Preferably, they should be prepared with water, coconut water, or plant-based milk and without added refined sugar. If available, choose for them to be sweetened with stevia or some other natural sweetener. (You can bring a stevia or monk fruit packet with you to sweeten your beverages.)

- If you are going to attend a party or social event, make sure that what you choose to eat is prepared as I recommended earlier. Desserts and pastries are better to avoid, as they usually contain refined sugars, dairy, and unhealthy fats. If you do not know what will be served at the event, it is recommended that you eat in advance at home. This way, you won't feel guilty about eating a full meal of things you shouldn't eat.

Final Thoughts on the Diet

It is important to clarify that the only way to obtain results by following this diet is if you are constant and follow it strictly for at least 90 days. However, not everything comes down to just following the diet described here, as it must be complemented with the other steps that we will mention later. You should also keep in mind that once this period of time passes, you cannot start eating anything you want without problems, even if you think that you are completely healed, as this is most likely not so. In most cases, the stomach lining will not be as strong as it was before you had gastritis, even after a year of feeling healed.

Another thing that I want to clarify is that although there are different types of gastritis, and that it is common to find people who suffer from the same type of gastritis, not all those who suffer from the same type of gastritis will have the same symptoms. This is because even if it is the same type of gastritis, it can manifest as mild, moderate, or severe. Thus, it is possible that some people have problems with some foods that are allowed in the diet, especially those people who have recently been diagnosed and have severe symptoms.

Therefore, taking into account the aforementioned, if you were recently diagnosed with gastritis and have very severe symptoms, or have been suffering from this problem for a long time but with very annoying symptoms, following a diet as described below for at least the first four or six weeks can be very helpful to establish a base healing. These are some of the key points to follow:

- Follow a low-fat, low-acid, and low-salt diet
- Avoid raw foods and all irritating foods and beverages
- Eat soft and easy-to-digest foods in small portions (cream of rice, purees, cooked vegetables, etc.)
- Decrease the consumption of animal protein (you can temporarily replace animal protein with hemp or pea protein powder)

It is possible that, following this type of diet, you will lose some weight at first. However, do not worry, as you can recover it. In Appendix C (at the end of the book), I have included some tips on how to gain weight. I recommend that you start following or applying these tips to gain weight after you have established a base healing or when your stomach begins to improve and you can tolerate more food.

Once the first 90 days have passed, you can start adding a new food to your diet every three or seven days. It is recommended that when adding a new food, you eat it for a few days and see how well you tolerate it. If you react to a food, return to eating foods that you tolerate for a couple of days before trying another new food. You can keep a food journal in which you write down when and how much you ate of a particular food. Then, using a scale from 1 to 10, write down how well you tolerated that food. You can write a 10 if you tolerated it well and without any problems and write a 0 if the food caused you a lot of stomach problems. This may seem like a lot of work and a bit frustrating but it will help you find out which foods you tolerate and which ones you do not.

Finally, if you do not feel comfortable adding new foods or have not improved enough, you can continue with the diet described in this first step as long as you think it is necessary for your stomach to recover. My only recommendation is that you do not limit your diet too much and always try to eat as varied as possible, focusing on the consumption of vegetables and fruits, as these contain anti-inflammatory substances and will provide you with the vitamins and minerals that your body needs.

SECOND STEP

Change Your Habits and Lifestyle

In the first step, we talked about what foods you should avoid and include in your diet during the first 90 days. In this second step, we will talk about the most common bad habits that negatively affect the stomach lining and about the changes you must make in your lifestyle to facilitate the recovery of your stomach.

First, we will talk about the bad habits that you should eliminate. Then I will give you some tips and recommendations that will help you treat your gastritis.

- **Do not skip meals.** It is important that you develop the habit of eating on time and avoid skipping meals. If you go many hours without eating, you will allow stomach acid and pepsin to come into direct contact with the stomach lining, which will give them the opportunity to cause more irritation and inflammation in your stomach. It is not enough to eat healthily; you also need a fixed schedule to do it. (We will talk about this later.) Avoiding the skipping of meals plays an important role in the prevention and cure of gastritis.

- **Don't drink water while eating.** When you drink a lot of water or any type of beverage with your food, you dramatically decrease the concentration of stomach acid and digestive enzymes. This, in turn, causes your stomach to produce more stomach acid to reacidify its contents and be able to correctly break down certain foods that require a more acidic environment (as is the case with animal protein). If you want to facilitate the swallowing of food, you can take small sips of water but never in large amounts. Staying hydrated is very important, as it takes a lot of water to create the mucous layer or mucosal barrier of the stomach. Therefore, it is recommended that you drink water at least 30 minutes before or two hours after eating.

- **Do not lie down after eating.** If you usually lie down or sleep immediately after eating, you should stop doing that. When you are in a reclined position, food and gastric juices move to the upper part of your stomach. This not only makes digestion difficult but can also cause both stomach acid and pepsin to rise into the esophagus, resulting in burning and inflammation. It is recommended that, after eating, you remain upright or walk for a while to help facilitate digestion. Also, wait at least three hours before going to sleep. Always sleep on the left side and raise the head of the bed about five or 10 inches to prevent gastric juices from rising into your esophagus while you sleep or lie down.

- **Do not smoke.** The nicotine in cigarettes increases gastric acid secretion, which, in turn, can cause more irritation and inflammation in your stomach.[8] In addition, smoking restricts the small blood vessels in the stomach, which causes a reduction in blood flow in the area and slows the healing process.

- **Do not take non-steroidal anti-inflammatory drugs.** As I mentioned earlier, nonsteroidal anti-inflammatory drugs such as ibuprofen, naproxen, diclofenac, aspirin, etc., damage the stomach lining and inhibit the synthesis of prostaglandins, which leaves the stomach lining susceptible to damage by irritating and corrosive substances. If you need something to eliminate or soothe any pain not related to gastritis, the only analgesic allowed and that you could use is paracetamol. However, it is better that you consult with your doctor before consuming it.

- **Do not eat very hot or very cold foods.** Another thing you should avoid doing is eating foods or drinks that are very hot or very cold. It is recommended that you consume your meals when they are warm and, in the case of beverages, just slightly cold. However, this also depends on everyone's tolerance and, possibly, on the type of gastritis from which you suffer. My recommendation is that if your symptoms are very severe or if you have a very sensitive stomach, you follow this advice as much as you can.

Now that you know some of the bad habits you should eliminate, we will talk about the five tips that I strongly recommend that you start following as part of your plan to treat gastritis.

Tip #1: Eat Small Meals

Instead of eating three large meals a day, it is better to divide them into about five smaller meals that you eat every two or three hours. When you overeat, it is much more difficult to carry out digestion, as the food stays longer inside your stomach, whose expansion causes more stomach acid to be released.[33] Therefore, by eating small meals throughout the day, you will avoid overloading your stomach, digestion will be carried out more easily, and blood flow to the stomach lining will increase, thus facilitating the recovery process.

A small meal can be a cup of vegetables, half a cup of rice, and a portion of chicken breast or fish that is smaller than the palm of your hand (three or four ounces). While some people suffering from gastritis tolerate the combination of proteins and concentrated carbohydrates (for example, chicken with rice or potatoes), for others, this can be a problem. Therefore, it is recommended that when you eat protein-rich foods (chicken, fish, eggs, etc.), you try not to combine them with an excessive amount of concentrated carbohydrates (potatoes, rice, sweet potatoes, etc.). Doing this will help you speed up the digestion of proteins, which is usually harder to carry out when you suffer from gastritis.

Although it may be beneficial for some people to avoid mixing carbohydrates with their high-protein meals, for others, it may not be at all, as eating only protein and vegetables at a meal can make you lose weight in the long term. Therefore, my recommendation is that you see if your digestion improves when you mix only cooked vegetables with protein-rich foods. If you feel that this is helping you digest your meals better, but at the same time is making you lose a lot of weight, try adding some carbohydrates to your main meals, though without going overboard (for example, half a cup of rice, potatoes, sweet potatoes, etc.). After all, the answer lies in listening to your body.

The following meal schedule will give you an idea of when you should eat a specific meal:

Breakfast	7:00 to 8:30 a.m.
Mid-morning	10:00 to 11:00 a.m.
Lunch	12:30 to 2:00 p.m.
Snack	4:00 to 5:00 p.m.
Dinner	6:00 to 7:30 p.m.

NOTE: Remember that you should not eat anything three hours before bedtime, nor drink any beverage at least one hour before bedtime.

Tip #2: Chew Food Well

Digestion is a very demanding task that requires a lot of energy, especially when the stomach is forced to digest improperly chewed food. That is why it is extremely important to develop the habit of chewing food well, as chewing your food not only will facilitate the task of digestion but also allow your stomach to break down the food faster and work more efficiently.

In a 1967 study, it was shown that chewing food well provides saliva with a greater buffering capacity against stomach acid and that mucin-rich saliva (the main component of salivary and mucous secretions) mixed with food strengthens the mucosal defense against stomach acid and irritating substances. Meanwhile, foods that are mixed with a little saliva or ingested with little or no chewing absorb less stomach acid.[69]

Now that you know that chewing is the first step of the digestion process, you should also know that chewing the food until it is practically liquefied in your mouth brings with it two other great benefits.

First, it ensures that food mixes well with saliva, which contains digestive enzymes that help break down food and further facilitate its digestion in the stomach and small intestine. One of these enzymes is lingual lipase, which is responsible for breaking down fats and is activated by the presence of an acidic pH (when it reaches the stomach). The other is lingual amylase, an enzyme that partially breaks down carbohydrates in the mouth (thus beginning their digestion), that is mostly active at a neutral pH (7.0), and that is inactivated once the stomach pH drops below 4. The viscous texture of saliva also allows lubrication of the bolus, which facilitates swallowing and the transit of food along the gastrointestinal tract.

Secondly, this helps the intestine absorb nutrients more easily and maximizes the calories obtained from food. The more you chew your food, the fewer nutrients will be lost and the more they can be absorbed. Some of the foods that I especially recommend that you chew very well (until they are well crumbled in your mouth) are chicken, turkey, fish, and any source of animal protein, as doing this will greatly facilitate the digestion of the same.

That is why, and for everything else mentioned above, it is important that you chew your food well and take your time to eat slowly and without haste. If you are stressed, it is recommended that you relax before you start eating and that while you are eating, you avoid being distracted by your cell phone, computer, or television. Being present in the moment, relaxed, and focused on what you are eating will help you eat slowly and chew food well. I know this requires retraining a lifelong habit, but it is absolutely essential that you chew your food (or each bite) three to five times more than normal.

Tip #3: Decrease Salt and Sugar Consumption

When consumed excessively, salt irritates the stomach lining.[70] Therefore, it is better to reduce salt intake as much as possible and to avoid eating salty foods. Replace refined salt with a less processed salt such as sea salt or Himalayan pink salt.

Sugar, which is an ingredient that has been present in our diet for many years, is currently seen as one of the worst ingredients in modern life. One of the main reasons for this change in perspective is the harmful effects that sugar has on our body and the fact that it increases the risk of obesity, diabetes, and heart disease. In addition, excessive sugar consumption causes intestinal permeability,[71] promotes inflammation within the body, and feeds the bad bacteria and opportunistic yeast (such as Candida albicans) that live in our intestinal tract.

The overgrowth of opportunistic bacteria and yeast often leads to a condition known as dysbiosis. This overgrowth displaces beneficial bacteria, causing changes in the intestinal mucus barrier. When this barrier contains less beneficial bacteria, the permeability of the intestine is altered, allowing large substances and particles to enter the bloodstream, which trigger inflammatory and immunological responses.

On the other hand, Candida albicans, a common yeast that usually lives within our digestive system, usually does not cause any problems, as our gut flora prevents its growth. However, when an imbalance occurs between the gut flora and the immune system, this yeast can multiply and grow excessively, resulting in a candida overgrowth. When this yeast seizes our intestines, it releases more toxins into the bloodstream, which negatively affects our nervous and immune systems. Candida can also anxiously ask you for sweets and carbohydrates, which feed it and contribute even more to its proliferation.

Therefore, it is important that you know that a diet high in refined sugar will only cause more inflammation within your body and will contribute to the overgrowth of bad bacteria and yeast such as Candida albicans.

However, the idea here is not that you get rid of sweeteners forever. Rather, I recommend that you replace refined sugar and artificial sweeteners with natural sweeteners such as stevia, pure maple syrup, monk fruit, or coconut sugar. (Use them in moderation.) To sweeten some recipes, you can use dates, too. Honey is another good natural sweetener but it has an average pH of 4, so if you have very severe symptoms, it is better to avoid consuming honey until you feel better. Alternatively, you can neutralize the acidity of honey by adding it to smoothies made with almond milk or use it to make marinades.

Tip #4: Exercise Regularly

Including an exercise session in your daily routine will be beneficial not only for your digestive system but for your overall health. An exercise session does not have to last for a long time; about 20 or 30 minutes is more than enough.

I recommend that you start walking for 15 or 20 minutes every day, preferably after eating, as this will help with the digestion process. Another thing that I recommend is that you avoid exercises that are very strenuous or that put a lot of pressure on your abdomen (for example, weightlifting, abdominal exercises, high-impact aerobics, gymnastics, or any activity that requires too much effort for your body).

If you regularly perform any of the activities mentioned above, you do not have to stop doing them. However, I recommend that you take note of any changes in your symptoms or of whether you notice that they get worse after you perform a specific activity or exercise.

It is also recommended that you avoid performing high-intensity exercises after eating. Preferably, wait at least two or three hours. The most important part is to pay attention to how you feel. If you realize that some activity or exercise worsens your symptoms, it is better that you stop doing it until you feel better.

Finally, after you start walking and your stomach symptoms improve, you can add other types of cardiovascular exercises to your routine; for example, use an exercise bike or elliptical, go swimming or jogging, or do moderate workout routines with your body weight.

Tip #5: Protect Your Stomach

Throughout this book, we have talked about how the stomach lining is constantly attacked by substances such as stomach acid, pepsin, and other irritants. We have also talked about how the defense mechanisms of the stomach work and how the stomach defends itself against most irritants.

However, when you suffer from gastritis, one of the most important things that you should do, and that is often overlooked (or not given enough importance), is to constantly protect your stomach lining. One of the reasons why it is important to do this is that when the stomach is inflamed, it is much more difficult for it to defend itself against most irritants. Therefore, to accelerate the healing process, you must constantly protect your stomach lining, as diet alone may not be enough for the stomach lining to recover.

To protect the stomach lining, you can use a drug with a gastroprotective effect, such as sucralfate. This medication not only protects the stomach lining, but also stimulates the production of gastroprotective agents such as gastric mucus, bicarbonate, and prostaglandins.[72] Research shows that this medication forms a barrier and coat the gastric lesion. This protects the gastric lesion from stomach acid, pepsin, and bile, allowing it to heal. This medication is the closest thing to a Band-Aid that you can use to protect your stomach lining, though you must take it often and correctly so that it can work effectively. It is preferable that you consult your doctor before you take this medication.

A natural alternative to sucralfate is deglycyrrhized licorice, better known as DGL. It is a standardized extract that retains many of the healing properties of licorice root but without the side effects (hypertension, edema, and headache) of glycyrrhizin, which is the main component of that root. The therapeutic effect of DGL stems from its ability to restore the integrity of the stomach and intestinal lining. It does this by stimulating the production of prostaglandins in the gastrointestinal tract, which increases the secretion of gastric mucus and other protective factors of the stomach and intestinal lining.[73] In addition, DGL has an added antioxidant action that contributes to its effectiveness.[74]

It is also important that you protect your stomach from nocturnal gastric acid secretion while you sleep, as the stomach content reaches its maximum acidity (gastric pH drops below 4) during deep sleep. Normally, nocturnal gastric acid secretion begins after midnight and ends in the early hours of the morning.[75] To protect your stomach lining while you sleep, you have two options.

The first option is to take a medication with a gastroprotective effect, such as sucralfate, before going to sleep. By forming a barrier, this can help protect the stomach lining (especially gastric lesions) for up to six hours. The other option is to take histamine H2 receptor blockers (such as famotidine or cimetidine), which may be a good option before you go to sleep, as they inhibit acid secretion for only about eight to 12 hours, without affecting acid secretion during the day.[76] Combined therapy of both medications can be much more effective than taking each medication separately.

Another medication that can be very effective in protecting your stomach lining is rebamipide, commercially known as Mucosta. The mechanism of action of this medication is through the stimulation of prostaglandins in the stomach lining.

This causes the stomach to produce gastric mucus and bicarbonate, thus accelerating the healing process.[77] In a study conducted in 2008, the efficacy of rebamipide therapy was evaluated in patients with chronic gastritis and symptoms of dyspepsia. At the end of the study, it was observed that all patients who underwent treatment with rebamipide saw a significant improvement in their gastric symptoms; there was also an improvement in the endoscopic and histological characteristics of the stomach linings of those patients.[78]

That said, while the medications mentioned above may be effective in helping you treat gastritis, it is recommended that you consult with your doctor before you start taking any of them.

Final Thoughts on the Habits and Lifestyle Changes

As I suggest in the first step, it is necessary that you also get rid of all the bad habits that we mentioned in this step and that you make the requisite changes in your lifestyle, so that your stomach can recover faster.

However, unlike the first step, it is recommended that you permanently eliminate (or avoid as much as possible) most of the habits that we mentioned throughout this step. Otherwise, more than likely, the symptoms or discomfort in the stomach will return, if you continue with the bad habits that contributed to your gastritis in the first place.

THIRD STEP

Manage Your Stress and Anxiety Levels

Previously, we talked about all the foods that you should avoid and those that you can consume in your diet, the bad habits that you should eliminate, and some changes that you should make in your lifestyle. In this third and final step, we will focus only on stress and mental health, as when it comes to treating gastritis, keeping stress under control is as important as following the proper diet or changing your bad eating habits and your lifestyle.

When you suffer from gastritis, stress is not the only thing that can prevent or make the recovery of your stomach more difficult. Anxiety can also prevent and slow down the healing process. Therefore, it is extremely important that you pay close attention to this step and not take it lightly. In most cases, stress and anxiety are the main reasons why people who suffer from gastritis never heal completely.

What is Stress?

We've all heard about stress and how bad it can be for our health but most people don't know what stress really is. In itself, stress is nothing more than a natural response or physiological reaction in which various defense mechanisms come into play to deal with situations that are perceived as threatening or challenging and that, to address, require a mobilization of physical, mental, and behavioral resources. Therefore, it can be said that stress is an adaptive and emergency process that protects us and helps us survive.

Although the word "stress" usually has a negative connotation, it is not all bad. In fact, stress can be both "good" and "bad."

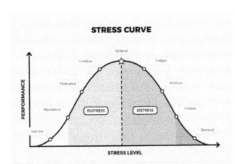

On the one hand, good or positive stress—better known as eustress—is a type of stress that stimulates and motivates us to face challenges or problems harmoniously and effectively. Eustress increases vitality and energy, facilitating decision-making. It can also be defined as a state of positive excitement that keeps us alert and allows us to be creative, take initiative, and respond efficiently to those situations that require it. This type of stress is temporary and does not cause anguish or anxiety.

Bad or negative stress, also known as distress, arises when we are unable to adapt to stressful situations or when we are overcome by the challenge or problem we are facing. As a result, due to the excessive and continuous use of our physical and mental resources, the body enters a state of tension, fatigue, and mental exhaustion, leading us to experience a lack of energy, irritability, nervousness, anxiety, anguish, panic attacks, insomnia, loss of appetite, stomach upset, tension headaches, and more.

It can be said that eustress and distress are two sides of the same coin or slopes of the same process. Let's see how stress is classified according to its duration:

- **Acute stress.** This occurs in the short term and does not last over time. It arises from the pressures and demands of something new or exciting happens, or due to emergency and dangerous situations that require a rapid reaction (for example, when you run or fight for your life in the face of a threat, when you suddenly press the brakes to avoid an accident, when you have an argument with someone or a day with a lot of work, etc.). It can be said that, initially, this is a kind of good or positive stress, though when it exceeds our ability to cope with the situation, it can become distress or negative stress. Due to its short duration, it does not cause significant damage to the body beyond anger, irritability, anxiety, tension headaches, stomach upset, or temporary overexcitation, which manifests itself in the form of an increase in blood pressure, a fast heartbeat, excessive perspiration, etc.

- **Chronic stress.** This occurs when negative stress is constant or persists for a long period of time and when the person perceives that they have little or no control over the situation. Negative stress becomes chronic when a person faces continuous challenges without relief or relaxation between stressors. The time can vary from several weeks to months. This type of stress can also be the result of traumatic events of the past that have been internalized and that always remain present as something painful or disturbing. The consequences of chronic stress are severe, particularly because it contributes to a more severe state of anxiety and depression. If it is not treated in time, chronic stress can cause other health problems that go beyond gastritis, such as the weakening of your immune system or an increased risk of having a heart attack or cardiovascular accident.[79]

Countless things can cause both acute and chronic stress. Because it is so individualized, the person who suffers from it is the one who can best identify its source. However, while it is true that stress can be caused by many things, it can be classified into two main sources:

•   **Internal stress.** This is what we create when we worry for no reason or about things we cannot control or do anything about. The way we see and perceive certain situations can cause us stress. Some examples are having irrational and pessimistic thoughts about life, speaking negatively about ourselves, setting unrealistic or negative expectations, always seeking perfection, or wanting to have control of everything. Negative emotions and thoughts can be more stressful than external stressful situations (which we will discuss next). This type of stress is one of the most important to understand and manage.

•   **External stress.** This is the one that stems from external situations or that does not come from our own thoughts and that, in some way or another, can interfere with our peace of mind. External stressors can include pressures we are subject to (either at work or at school), responsibilities at home, unexpected situations or events such as the loss of a loved one or of a job, a breakup or a divorce, economic or family problems, traffic on the way to work or home, etc. This may be one of the most difficult types of stress to avoid because many people feel that it is beyond their control.

Sometimes what causes internal or external stress depends, at least in part, on how you perceive it, as what can generate negative stress in one person may not stress another person. For example, having to face traffic on the way to work can be stressful for you, as you may worry that traffic will make you late, while for other people, it can be a trip they can enjoy listening to music while driving. Therefore, it can be said that, often, the way we perceive and react to certain situations at the subconscious level is more harmful to our health than a stressful event over which we have no control.

Stress and Your Body

Now that you know what stress is, we will talk in depth about what happens in the body when we are stressed. When we get stressed, two main hormones are released in our body: cortisol and adrenaline. Both are known as the "stress hormones" and are produced by the adrenal glands, which are located just above the kidneys.

When we feel fear or perceive danger, a response in our body known as "fight or flight" is automatically activated. This causes adrenaline and cortisol to be released into the bloodstream, preparing us to face the situation or threat. The release of these hormones causes a series of internal reactions such as increased heart rate, respiratory rate, and blood pressure, as well as the decrease or inhibition of digestion, reproduction, growth, and immunity. The latter are unnecessary bodily functions during the stress situation.[79] The body makes these physical changes to increase your strength, boost the speed of your reaction time, and improve your focus.

In the past, this state of alert helped our ancestors survive in an aggressive, dangerous, and hostile environment. Every day was a challenge for them, as they had to get resources to survive. The nights were dark and wild animal attacks were frequent.

In that situation, stress was not negative; it was essential for survival, as our ancestors had to be constantly alert. Therefore, it can be said that positive stress helped our ancestors be faster, be stronger, and have more reflexes.

While it is true that, currently, we do not usually adopt a maximum alert response or reaction, as man did in prehistoric times, we do operate as if we were in a state of constant and a low degree of emergency due to the demands and pressures of modern life.

Adrenaline and cortisol are not the only hormones that are released in your body when you are stressed. Norepinephrine, glucagon, and prolactin are other hormones involved in stress processes.[80] Most of these hormones are essential for coping with and responding to stressful situations. However, when their levels are very high (especially cortisol), they can negatively impact our health.

The stress response has a lot to do with the autonomic nervous system, which is the part of the nervous system that controls and regulates internal organs such as the stomach, intestines, and heart, without the need for a conscious effort by the body. The nervous system is divided into different subsystems, among which the sympathetic and parasympathetic nervous systems stand out, with opposite functions. Next, we will talk about each of these systems and the roles they play in the human body.

Sympathetic System

This is the system that prepares the body to react to a stressful situation and that predominates when there is both positive and negative stress. (The degree of activation depends on the level of stress.) This system is the one that is responsible for the "fight or flight" response and that causes, through the adrenal glands, the release of adrenaline, norepinephrine, and cortisol in the bloodstream, to prepare the body to deal with the stressful situation.[81] Some of the responses for which the sympathetic nervous system is responsible are:

- Acceleration of heart and respiratory rate
- Increased blood pressure and blood flow to the muscles
- Dilation of the bronchial tubes and pupils
- Excessive sweating
- Stimulation of the adrenal glands to release adrenaline, norepinephrine, and cortisol
- Blood glucose release from the liver
- Suppression of the immune system
- Reduction or slowdown of digestion and peristaltic contractions

Parasympathetic System

Unlike the previous system, the parasympathetic system is responsible for regulating and decelerating the body, allowing it to return to a state of rest after a period of stress or energy expenditure.[81] The main nerve, and one of the most important of this system, is the vagus nerve, as this and the neurotransmitter acetylcholine regulate all the internal organs that are affected by the activation of the sympathetic system.[82] Some of the functions that the parasympathetic system carries out are:

- Decreasing the heart and respiratory rate
- Reducing the blood pressure
- Contracting the bronchial tubes and pupils
- Relaxing the muscles
- Stimulating digestion and digestive secretions
- Increasing peristaltic activity

- Repairing tissue and boosting immune activity

The autonomic nervous system is not only divided into these two systems just mentioned, as the enteric nervous system is also part of it. The enteric nervous system is made up of networks of millions of neurons found in the tissues that line the esophagus, stomach, small intestine, and colon, which are some of the organs that are part of the digestive system. Likewise, this system independently regulates all the vital functions of the digestive system—that is, it does not need the brain to tell them what to do.[83] It also receives signals from the sympathetic and parasympathetic nervous system and communicates with the brain (or central nervous system) through the vagus nerve.

Returning to the issue of stress, what we know as stress is nothing more than an imbalance between the sympathetic and parasympathetic systems caused by sustained tension. Therefore, to recover the balance between both systems, the activation of the parasympathetic system can be resorted through the stimulation of the vagus nerve and other techniques that help relax the mind and body.

Before we go into detail about what you can do to stimulate the vagus nerve and relax both your mind and your body, let's move on to the next part and learn a little about the relationship between anxiety and gastritis.

Anxiety and Gastritis

Anxiety appears mostly when we cannot adapt to stressful situations, though sometimes it can appear even when we have not been subjected to any type of stressful situation that we can identify. Although there are many types of anxiety, each with different causes, in terms of gastritis, the most common type is anxiety due to nutritional deficiencies, a gut flora imbalance, or pain and stomach discomfort caused by inflammation and irritation of the stomach lining.[23,84,85]

On the one hand, deficiencies of Vitamin D, magnesium, the B vitamins (particularly B12, B6, and folate), zinc, iron, selenium, omega-3 fatty acids, and amino acids can cause anxiety, depression, sudden changes in mood, and other problems related to mental health.[86,87] Therefore, the first step you should take to treat anxiety (and depression) is to find out in which of those nutrients you might be deficient. I recommend that you go to a doctor, either a naturopath or functional, so he or she can help you get tested for nutritional deficiencies.

Addressing those nutrient deficiencies will not only help you reduce anxiety but also increase your ability to properly manage stress. Often, deficiencies in these nutrients are due to poor nutrition or the prolonged use of antacid medications. The latter does not allow your body to properly absorb a large number of minerals and vitamins,[88] and can cause anxiety and depression as a side effect.[89]

On the other hand, an imbalance in the microbiota or gut flora (something that is usually common when you suffer from gastritis) can cause anxiety, depression, and mood swings.[85] However, the imbalance in the gut flora and nutritional deficiencies are not the only causes of anxiety and depression when one is suffering from gastritis, as both disorders can also be caused by the same disease. For example, you can experience anxiety when you feel a lot of discomfort or pain in the stomach, either because the stomach lining is very irritated or inflamed, because of the constant concern that something bad may happen, or because you are obsessed with your symptoms.

Scientific evidence shows that there is bidirectional communication between the digestive system and the brain—called the gut-brain axis—which is carried out through neural (vagus nerve), endocrine (HPA axis), and immune (cytokine).[90] Therefore, any imbalance in your stomach or intestine might make you feel anxious, depressed, or even fatigued.[23]

Considering that an imbalance in the gut flora is usually common with gastritis, improving your digestive health will help alleviate or eliminate the symptoms of anxiety or depression that you may be experiencing. For this, you will need to balance your gut flora with the help of probiotics (which we will talk about in the next chapter) and reduce inflammation in both the stomach and intestine.

Tips for Reducing Stress and Anxiety

Throughout this third step, we have talked about what stress is, what substances are released in the body when we are stressed, the close relationship between anxiety and gastritis, and how stress and thoughts or emotions can negatively affect you overall health. In this last part, we will talk only about the things you can do to reduce or manage your stress and anxiety levels.

Although countless techniques can help you reduce stress, when it comes to treating it, the first and most important thing to do is identify what causes you stress. Then see how you can deal with that situation or the things that stress you. Often, family, school, work, relationships, money, and health are the main sources of stress for most people. The way to deal with these external stressors is to change how you perceive them in order to change how you respond to them and how much they affect you emotionally, physically, and mentally.

Therefore, it is important that you become aware of the things that cause you stress and ask yourself why you should stress out about them. For example, you may feel emotionally bad about being sick. However, instead of emphasizing the problem, you should focus on the solution and think about what you need to do to heal. Negative thoughts will not help you recover, so my first recommendation is to be positive and maintain an optimistic attitude.

Supplements

Many natural supplements have proven to be effective in treating anxiety, mitigating the negative effects of stress and reducing cortisol levels. However, because the list is quite extensive, I will speak only of the natural supplements that have proven (through research and clinical trials) to be the most effective at reducing stress and treating anxiety.

While the natural supplements that we will mention below can help you treat anxiety and increase your resistance to stress, it is recommended that you make sure you meet your essential nutrient needs, as both stress and anxiety consume and deplete vitamins and minerals. Therefore, if you have been suffering from chronic stress or anxiety for a long time, you may have nutritional deficiencies that are worsening your anxiety or preventing your body from managing stress properly.

Some of these essential nutrients are minerals such as magnesium and zinc; vitamins such as C, D, and B (especially B6, B12, and folic acid); omega-3 fatty acids; and certain amino acids. The latter are neurotransmitter precursors and are necessary for the proper functioning of the nervous system.[91] In particular, Vitamin B6 is essential for the formation of the neurotransmitters GABA, serotonin, and dopamine.[92] GABA is known as the brain chemical of relaxation, serotonin as the substance of happiness, and dopamine as a neurotransmitter that helps you stay focused and motivated.

These three neurotransmitters have a strong impact on mood. It is also important that you keep your magnesium levels in the healthy range, as this mineral helps relax the nervous system, stabilizes the mood, and can effectively combat anxiety.[93]

Now that you know about the importance of satisfying your basic nutritional needs, let's look at natural supplements that can help you treat anxiety and reduce your stress levels.

Rhodiola Rosea

This is an adaptogenic herb, also known as golden root or arctic root, that has been used for years in traditional Chinese medicine and Scandinavian countries to increase energy, improve mood, and increase resistance to physical and mental stress. Rhodiola rosea helps balance the stress response system, thereby reducing anxiety and excessive emotional reactivity, which allows the person to remain calmer and cope better with the stressful situation.[94] One of the ways in which this herb works is by increasing the activity of the neurotransmitters serotonin and dopamine in the brain and of opioids such as beta-endorphins.[95] One of the most studied benefits of Rhodiola rosea is that it helps people deal with chronic or prolonged fatigue.[96]

Some studies have shown that Rhodiola rosea helps treat both mild and moderate depression and generalized anxiety disorders.[97,98] So, if you usually get very stressed or suffer from fatigue, depression, or anxiety, Rhodiola rosea is a natural alternative you should consider. The Rhodiola rosea supplement you choose must be standardized to contain at least 3% rosavins and 1% salidroside, which are the main components that confer the therapeutic benefits of this herb.

The recommended average dose is around 500 mg, although because it is a bit stimulating, Rhodiola rosea should be taken early in the day so that it does not interrupt your sleep. This herb can interact with antidepressant medications, so you should not take it if you are on such medications.[99] Consult with a naturopath or functional doctor before you start taking this supplement.

Ashwagandha

This is another effective adaptogenic herb, known as Indian ginseng, which has been used for centuries in Ayurvedic medicine to treat anxiety and help people adapt to stress.[100] A very interesting benefit related to this herb is its ability to help you achieve a restful sleep, which is very useful when you suffer from exhaustion caused by stress.[101] Ashwagandha helps reduce prolonged stress through the stimulation of GABA receptors and serotonin in the brain, thus producing a relaxing effect on the body.[100]

Although the benefits of Ashwagandha are multiple, one of the most interesting is its impact on the stress hormone cortisol. In studies conducted with people suffering from chronic stress, it was found that Ashwagandha reduced blood cortisol levels by over 25%.[102] When it comes to reducing cortisol, Ashwagandha is one of the most effective adaptogenic herbs. The key to its effectiveness lies in the alkaloids and steroid lactones, called ananolides, which help normalize a wide range of biochemical functions.

The average dose is 300-500 mg standardized to contain at least 2 to 5% of ananolides, once or twice a day. This herb has a mild sedative effect, so it is preferable to consume it at night. It is not recommended for pregnant women or if you are taking anxiolytic or antidepressant medications. If, when you start to take it, you experience stomach discomfort, discontinue its use. Consult with a naturopath or functional doctor before you start taking this supplement.

L-Theanine

This is a rare amino acid considered a natural anxiolytic because it produces a calming effect on the brain and induces a mental state described as "calm attention" or "focused relaxation." It is not commonly found in the human diet and it does not belong to the group of essential and non-essential amino acids. This amino acid is found mostly in green, black, white, and oolong tea.

This amino acid produces a calming effect by crossing the blood-brain barrier, thus causing greater activity of alpha brain waves and a greater synthesis of GABA.[103] The increase in GABA, in turn, increases the brain's levels of dopamine and serotonin, which produces a feeling of calm and well-being.

L-theanine is found almost exclusively in black, green, white, and oolong tea. Therefore, it should be consumed as a supplement, as both green and black tea contain caffeine, which can irritate the stomach lining and exacerbate gastritis symptoms.

The recommended dose of L-Theanine is 200 to 400 mg, once or twice a day. Unlike benzodiazepines and other medications for anxiety, L-theanine does not cause drowsiness; nor does it decrease reflexes or concentration. There are also no risks of developing a tolerance or dependence when L-theanine is taken for long periods of time.[104] So, it can be said that the consumption of L-theanine is safe for treating anxiety. Just keep in mind that this supplement may interact with other supplements or medications, especially those that lower the blood pressure. Therefore, it is recommended that you consult a naturopath or functional doctor before you start taking this supplement.

Other Supplements and Herbs

Many other supplements and natural herbs can help you treat both anxiety and stress. For example, there are many relaxing herbs to calm the nerves and relieve anxiety. Some of these herbs are valerian, passiflora, lemon balm, chamomile, lavender, gotu kola, and kava kava. While they can act in different ways according to their compounds and active ingredients, most of these relaxing herbs work, in part, by increasing GABA, which is the brain's calming chemical.

The interesting thing about these herbs is that to obtain their benefits, you do not have to consume them in the form of supplements, as you can prepare teas with them. However, while such relaxing herbs can help you calm anxiety, they do not help your body adapt to anxiety or prolonged stress the way that adaptogens herbs do.

With respect to adaptogenic herbs, it is important that you know that Rhodiola rosea and Ashwagandha are not the only herbs of this type that exist; bacopa, ginkgo biloba, ginseng panax, tulsi, and schisandra are also considered adaptogenic herbs. What most adaptogens have in common is that they help your body adapt better to physical and mental stress. Some herbs have more marked properties than others in terms of treating specific problems such as fatigue, concentration, depression, and anxiety. Therefore, when choosing an adaptogenic herb, you should opt for one whose benefits best match the symptoms from which you are suffering.

Finally, do not forget to consult with a naturopath or functional doctor before you start taking any of the supplements or herbs mentioned above.

Relaxation Techniques

Another very effective way to reduce stress and anxiety is with the help of relaxation techniques. In itself, a relaxation technique is any method or activity that helps reduce physical or mental stress. While there are many relaxation techniques, it is recommended that you start with one and practice it for a while. If you feel that it does not work, try another.

You can use the following relaxation techniques when you feel stressed or anxious, though it is recommended that you practice some of these techniques daily to increase your resistance to stress and anxiety. It is also convenient for you to practice them in a quiet and preferably secluded place.

Diaphragmatic Breathing

The first technique I will talk about is deep diaphragmatic breathing, also known as belly breathing, as it is a very easy technique to learn and do. You can practice this exercise at any time and in any place to stimulate your vagus nerve almost instantaneously. This, in turn, will activate the relaxation response and decrease the overactivation in your body caused by stress or anxiety.[82,105] The relaxation response, which is the opposite of the stress response, is necessary for healing, repair, and renewal processes in your body.

Another benefit of diaphragmatic breathing is that it allows you to consciously correct the mistakes we usually make when breathing. Most people breathe in the wrong way (chest breathing instead of belly breathing), which does not sufficiently oxygenate the blood. In themselves, breathing exercises are the basis of many other relaxation techniques. Therefore, if you have never done breathing or relaxation exercises, I recommend that you start with this exercise. To perform this breathing exercise, follow these steps:

- Sit in a comfortable place or lie on your back (on the bed or on a flat surface). Place one hand on your chest and another on your abdomen.
- Breathe slowly and deeply through your nose for four seconds. (You can count the time in your head.) While doing this, try to bring the air you inspire into the abdomen area, so that the hand on the abdomen moves slightly and the hand placed on your chest remains as still as possible.
- Hold the air for about three seconds (without any effort or pressure).
- Exhale slowly through the mouth with pursed lips (almost closed, as if you were inflating a balloon) for eight seconds. You must expel all the air. As you do it, you should feel your abdomen sinking or contracting.
- Keep your lungs empty for a second or two and then take a deep breath again, bringing the air back into your abdomen.
- Practice this breathing technique for five to 10 minutes, several times a day.

Performing this exercise even when you are not stressed, anxious, or nervous will help you acquire more practice on your breathing, which, in turn, will help you replace a quick breath with a slow one. Thus, you will achieve physical relaxation with a state of greater calm and serenity. At first, breathing in this way might seem a little weird and you may do it incorrectly. However, it will be only a matter of time and practice before you master this technique. Once you do, you won't need to place your hands on your chest or abdomen, as the movement will be more natural for you.

Meditation

Another very effective way to reduce stress and anxiety and to calm the mind is to practice meditation. Meditation is an ancient practice that has gained popularity in recent decades, mostly because of the benefits it has in terms of mental and emotional well-being. In addition, it has been shown that meditation increases vagal tone and parasympathetic activity in the body, leading your body and mind to a state of relaxation.[82]

Before we start talking about what you should do to start meditating, it is important that you know that there are many types of meditation.

Here, we will talk only about mindfulness meditation, which is an adaptation of traditional Buddhist meditation. Mindfulness consists of paying attention or being aware of what you are doing or feeling in the present moment. It is intended to avoid all kinds of worries, judgments, guilt, or thoughts of the past or future. Mindfulness supports and enriches meditation, while meditation nourishes and expands mindfulness. These are the steps to follow to practice this type of meditation:

• Find a quiet and secluded place. Sit in a chair, on the floor, or wherever you feel comfortable, with your head, neck, and back straight but not rigid. If you want, you can play relaxing background music, such as the sound of ocean waves or a waterfall.

• Close your eyes and become aware of your breathing. Focus on the sensations that emerge from it without trying to modify them in any way. Feel the sensation of the air entering and leaving your lungs while you breathe. Pay attention to the way you breathe and how your diaphragm expands.

• Observe how thoughts appear, whether from the past or the future. As they appear, try to put them aside and focus on breathing.

• If you get carried away by your thoughts, observe where your mind is going, without judging, and simply refocus on your breathing. Don't be hard on yourself when this happens to you.

• Do this as many times as necessary. Every time a thought comes, let it go and don't get involved with it. One trick is that you see your thoughts as clouds that come and go.

Like the previous relaxation technique, you may initially find it difficult to meditate but it will be only a matter of time and practice before you get used to it. The duration of the meditation depends on you and how much time you can dedicate to it. Ideally, start with five minutes and gradually increase. Once you have acquired the habit, you can devote 20 to 30 minutes daily to meditation, preferably in the morning. If you find it difficult to follow the above steps, I recommend that you look online for videos or audios about mindfulness meditation and then use them as a guide.

Other Techniques

There are other, more advanced relaxation techniques such as yoga, guided imagery, progressive muscle relaxation, autogenous relaxation, and tapping (emotional release technique), which I would like to talk about. However, because they are a bit complicated to explain in written words, I decided not to include them. If you are interested in any of these relaxation techniques, I recommend that you seek the help of a professional or therapist who is familiar with them, so they can guide you and teach you how to perform them correctly.

However, you don't really need the help of a professional, as if you take a look online, you will find videos and guided audios on how to perform these relaxation techniques.

Just remember that relaxation techniques are skills that require practice. As with any skill, your ability to relax will improve only if you practice. Be patient with yourself and don't let the effort you make to practice relaxation techniques become another stress factor.

Other Recommendations

Apart from the supplements and relaxation techniques mentioned above, you can make some changes to your lifestyle that can help you reduce stress and cortisol levels. The following tips and recommendations can help you not only manage your stress but also improve your mood and emotional well-being. So, I recommend that you follow them or include them in your daily routine.

- **Get enough sleep.** You need to get enough sleep so that your body can recover and better handle any stressful situation. Lack of sleep increases blood cortisol levels and leads to cognitive problems.[106] Therefore, for your body and mind to remain in good condition, it is recommended that you go to bed early and try to sleep at least seven hours every night. However, the amount of sleep you get is not the only thing that matters, as the quality of sleep is just as important as the number of hours you sleep. Some things you can do to improve the quality of your sleep is to go to bed at the same time every day, not eat three hours before going to sleep, and suppress any source of light in your room (for example, electronic devices or light coming from the street). If you find it difficult to fall asleep, try meditating or reading before sleeping.

- **Exercise.** Physical activity is an excellent way to combat stress and anxiety. One of the ways in which exercise reduces stress and anxiety is through the release of endorphins—also known as happiness hormones—in the brain. These can lead you to experience a general feeling of well-being.[107] Exercise can also improve your sleep quality, which can sometimes be adversely affected by stress and anxiety. However, although exercise may be good for you, you should avoid doing it in excess, as overtraining or performing very strenuous exercises can increase cortisol levels in the bloodstream. Therefore, it is recommended that you perform low-effort physical activities, such as walking. Start walking for 15 to 20 minutes three times a week and then for 30 minutes every day. Mind and body exercises such as yoga, tai chi, and qi gong are also very good for relieving stress.

- **Stop overthinking.** Keeping your mind occupied with tasks that require your attention and that do not bore you can be very useful techniques for avoiding overthinking and cutting the cycle of negative thoughts. This may seem like a very obvious piece of advice but forcing yourself to do or work on something while you're worried can prevent you from overthinking or cause your thoughts of worry to disappear. You can read a book, draw, sing, play an instrument, or do something you like that doesn't cause you more stress or anxiety. Doing something you enjoy helps promote a more conscious and meditative state of mind, which is useful for keeping your mind from constantly thinking about things in the past or future. The key here is not only to get yourself busy but to also, while you are engaging in any task or activity, pay attention to and be aware of what you are doing.

- **Spend time with positive people.** Surround yourself and spend time with people who support you and who are positive, as this can greatly help reduce your stress levels. Research has shown that when a person has social and emotional support (from friends or family), they tend to have lower cortisol levels.[108] This is because, during contact and social bonding, the hormone oxytocin is released; this can decrease anxiety and block increases in cortisol.[109] Therefore, if you lack friends, it is important that you make new friends—people with whom you can go out, laugh, and have fun. Although you may not want to be surrounded by other people when you feel sick to your stomach, making new friends can be one of the best things you do to avoid feeling alone or getting so involved in the disease.

- **Spend more time outside.** Something else that, apart from helping you deal with stress, can be very beneficial for your emotional well-being is spending more time outside. A growing number of studies have shown that visiting green spaces and being in touch with nature can not only help you reduce stress and cortisol levels but also improve your mood and increase feelings of happiness and well-being.[110,111]

- To experience this, you don't necessarily have to go out for hours or take a vacation. Simply spare 20 or 30 minutes of your day for walking or sitting in a place that makes you feel in touch with nature. After all, the important thing is to go out and not spend so much time at home or isolated from the world.

Other things you can do to reduce stress are to receive acupuncture sessions or full-body massages at least once a week. Listening to music can also have a very relaxing effect on the body—and even more so when it is combined with non-strenuous dances.

Final Thoughts on Stress and Anxiety

It is necessary for you to keep stress and anxiety under control, since, as we mentioned at the beginning of this step, both can make stomach recovery much more difficult. That is why learning to manage stress and having good emotional health is just as important as following a proper diet or eliminating bad habits and changing your lifestyle. Doing all these things together will create the kind of synergy that allows healing of the stomach to take place. I would now like to recap what we have talked about throughout this step about stress and anxiety.

The first thing you should do with respect to stress is to identify the situations that cause you stress. Then determine what you can do to avoid them. Once you have identified the cause or your stressors, you should become aware of why you react to stress the way you do, or how you perceive what causes you stress. Ask yourself why you should stress about something or allow it to affect you emotionally. Being aware of the way you react to certain situations will help you use the power of your mind to more quickly relax your body and mind. Meditation, diaphragmatic breathing, and yoga can be very useful in helping you reduce the stress of everyday life, as can the supplements and recommendations we talked about earlier.

However, another type of approach is needed to treat anxiety, as when you suffer from gastritis, it does not always have an associated stress factor. Often, nutritional deficiencies have a lot to do with anxiety. Thus, it is recommended that you start looking for deficiencies in some of the vitamins, minerals, or other nutrients that we mentioned in the part in which we talked about anxiety and gastritis.

Gastritis alone can generate anxiety, creating a vicious circle in which the anxiety caused by gastritis makes your stomach worse, which, in turn, generates more anxiety and increasingly fuels this vicious circle. There are two main routes to break the vicious circle of anxiety caused by gastritis. The first is to take some of the natural supplements to treat the anxiety we mentioned earlier. The other is to take anxiolytic medications.

While anxiolytic medications can be of great help in treating anxiety caused by gastritis, the side effects they may cause should be taken into account. For example, benzodiazepines are usually highly addictive; when you try to quit them, they can cause withdrawal symptoms and make you feel significantly worse than you felt before you started taking them.[112] Another side effect of benzodiazepines is that they can loosen the lower esophageal sphincter, causing or aggravating acid reflux.[113] An alternative to these could be selective serotonin reuptake inhibitors; they are not considered addictive and they do not relax the lower esophageal sphincter.

The consumption of such drugs should always be monitored or supervised by a healthcare professional, as the abuse or misuse of these drugs can make the situation worse and cause other problems.

Finally, it is important that you know that, in some cases, stress and anxiety can be caused by psychological trauma, when the person constantly remembers some traumatic situation or event that generates negative thoughts, feelings of guilt, anger, pain, etc.

If you feel that this could be the case with you, look for a psychologist to help you identify and treat those unresolved internal problems that may be causing psychological or emotional stress. A skilled cognitive behavioral therapist will know what to do and teach you how to modify your thoughts and emotions, as well as how to develop behaviors that help you deal with emotional problems with a more positive attitude.

Conclusion of the Healing Program

In the previous steps, we talked in depth about the diet you should follow, the bad eating habits that most affect the stomach lining, and how stress and anxiety affect it and make the recovery process almost impossible. In conclusion, I would like to talk about some things that will help you increase your chances of success by following this healing program.

My first recommendation is that you treat any nutritional deficiencies that you might have, specifically of certain vitamins and minerals that support the healing process, such as zinc and antioxidant vitamins such as A, C, and E. Zinc is very important for digestive health, as this mineral supports the integrity of the gastrointestinal lining and has antioxidant and anti-inflammatory properties.[114] Meanwhile, antioxidant vitamins such as A, C, and E fight free radicals and help reduce inflammation.

While deficiencies in these vitamins are usually not common, it is recommended that you at least maintain optimal levels or adequate consumption of foods that are rich in these vitamins. When you suffer from gastritis, you should also consume certain vitamins and minerals in forms that do not irritate your stomach lining. (We will talk more about this in Chapter 4.)

Linoleic acid deficiency is another nutritional deficiency that is often overlooked. However, treating it can be very helpful when one is suffering from gastritis.

This essential fatty acid of the omega-6 series is a precursor of prostaglandin E2, which increase the production of gastric mucus and bicarbonate and exert protective effects against the harmful actions of a large number of ulcerative agents. Therefore, it is recommended that you increase your consumption of foods rich in linoleic acid (or that you add to your treatment a supplement rich in gamma-linolenic acid), as this will increase the resistance of your stomach to stomach acid and pepsin. Don't forget to add to your diet foods rich in omega-3 fatty acids to maintain an adequate balance between the amount of omega-6 and omega-3 that you consume.

Another thing I recommend is that, together with your doctor, you try to find the root cause of your gastritis or what may be contributing to the inflammation in your stomach. While stomach acid and pepsin are often the main substances that irritate the stomach lining and keep it inflamed, there are other causes that may be affecting this vicious circle or that might be the main causes of inflammation in your stomach. These include Helicobacter pylori infection, viral infections that attack the stomach, bile reflux, among others.

On the other hand, if you were recently diagnosed with gastritis, it is possible that your doctor may have prescribed you inhibitors of gastric acid secretion, such as omeprazole and similar medications. Although these types of medications can help your stomach recover faster, they are not entirely a solution if the condition is chronic because a) they do not really treat the root cause of the problem and b) they can cause a series of complications if they are consumed for a long time, such as deficiencies in vitamins like B12 and folic acid and deficiencies in minerals such as magnesium, zinc, iron, and calcium.[88] In addition, long-term consumption of these medications can cause intestinal dysbiosis.[115] However, this does not mean that you should not take them; at the beginning, it might be a good idea to take them for about two or four weeks to calm the irritation in your stomach lining while you are following the diet and doing the other things that we have talked about in this healing program.

Finally, I recommend that you see the changes that you will make in your diet and habits as a new lifestyle that you are adopting, and that you do not worry so much about the fact that you are sick or obsessed with your symptoms. The simple act of worrying about the need to be very careful with every little thing you put in your mouth (out of fear of causing more damage to your stomach) will contribute to the idea that you are "sick" and that you cannot live "normally" like everyone else.

If you think you're going to get sick after eating a certain food that you shouldn't have, this is very likely to happen. I know that doing this is difficult when you feel very sick or have symptoms that do not let you live in peace but seeing everything in this way is the key for your stomach to recover faster. If you become obsessed with your symptoms or constantly think about the disease, you will feed the fear and possible anxiety you already have. Therefore, do not focus on the disease; the more you are aware of it and its symptoms, the harder it will be for your stomach to recover.

What If Symptoms Persist?

If symptoms persist 90 days after you started following the advice and recommendations of this healing program, it would be a good idea to review each of the above steps to see if you properly applied the most important points. Below, you will find a questionnaire about each of the most important points of this healing program.

Diet
• Did you eliminate from your diet all the irritating foods and drinks that we mentioned in the first step?
• Do the foods you eat daily come from the list of foods with a pH higher than 5? In the case of consuming acidic fruits, did you properly neutralize their acidity?
• Did you introduce into your diet foods that help combat inflammation of the stomach lining (such as flavonoid-rich foods)? If so, are you consuming enough of them daily?
• Did you introduce foods rich in linoleic acid into your diet (or did you add a supplement rich in gamma-linolenic acid to your treatment plan) to increase prostaglandin production? If so, did you also introduce foods rich in omega-3 to balance your intake of omega-6 fatty acids?
• Is the amount of fat you consume at each meal moderate (less than 15 grams of fat) or excessive (more than 15 grams of fat)? It is preferable that you consume less than 10 grams of fat per meal.
• Do you have an adequate intake of protein-rich foods to help repair the damaged tissues of your stomach?
• Are you eating only foods of soft consistency, foods that are easy to chew, and foods that are cooked and not raw?

Habits and Lifestyle
• Did you eliminate all the bad habits in the second step that can exacerbate inflammation in your stomach?
• Are you eating smaller portions of meals instead of large meals and are you dividing your main meals into five smaller ones so that you eat every three hours?
• Are you chewing each bite of food three to five times more than usual or until it is well crumbled in your mouth?
• Did you decrease the amount of salt you add to your meals and have you been avoiding very salty foods?

- Did you reduce your consumption of sugar and replace refined sugar and artificial sweeteners with healthier sweeteners such as stevia, pure maple syrup, monk fruit, etc.?
- Are you constantly protecting your stomach from gastric juices with a medication or supplement that has gastroprotective properties? If so, are you also protecting your stomach from nocturnal gastric acid secretion while you sleep?

Stress, Anxiety, and Emotional Wellbeing

- Did you identify that situation(s) that cause you stress? If so, did you do something about it or did you create a plan to manage your stress levels and keep stress at bay?
- If you suffer from anxiety, did you identify what causes that anxiety? If so, did you do something about it or did you create a plan to reduce your anxiety levels?
- Are you sleeping or resting enough to help your body handle stress better and recover faster?
- Are you engaging in physical activities to reduce your stress levels?
- Are you keeping your mind occupied with daily tasks or activities that require your attention, to avoid stressing yourself out by overthinking?
- Are you spending more time outside or going out to have fun with friends or family?

The idea is that if the symptoms persist, you should ask yourself all these questions to find out if there is any advice or if there are any recommendations that you are not applying, which may be preventing your stomach from recovering faster.

CHAPTER 4:BOOSTING THE HEALING PROCESS

In the previous chapter, we talked in depth about the three main steps of the healing program. However, there is also a fourth step, which was not included as such but that is undoubtedly the step that, once you start following and correctly applying the other steps, will help you speed up the recovery process of your stomach lining. I have dedicated this fourth chapter to talking about the fourth and last step, which consists of the most-used remedies and supplements for treating gastritis and its symptoms.

Because your stomach lining is inflamed (and, surely, it has been suffering for a long time), you must be patient once you start taking any of the remedies or supplements that we will talk about in this chapter, as they are not entirely "magical" and should be seen only as a means of supporting or aiding the recovery process of your stomach.

The following remedies and supplements were selected primarily for their gastroprotective, anti-inflammatory, and regenerative effects on the stomach lining, which have been proven through research and clinical studies conducted in recent years. Not all of the remedies and supplements that you find below will work the same or be effective for all people or all types of gastritis. Thus, you may have to try several of these until you find the one that works best for you.

Supplements for Gastritis

DGL (Deglycyrrhized Licorice)

DGL, also known as deglycyrrhized licorice, is a standardized extract of licorice root, which is typically used in the treatment of stomach complaints, including heartburn and indigestion. In the process of extracting DGL, glycyrrhizin is almost completely eliminated. This substance is responsible for many of the side effects of licorice, such as increased blood pressure (hypertension), fluid retention (swelling), the reduction of potassium levels, and headaches. The low levels of this substance make this supplement safe for long-term use.

Research has shown that DGL has the ability to increase the production of prostaglandins in the endothelial cells of the stomach, which results in an increase in the secretion of gastric mucus, bicarbonate, and other defense mechanisms of the stomach lining.[73] It has also been shown that several flavonoids found in the DGL have bactericidal properties against Helicobacter pylori and have important anti-inflammatory, antioxidant, and antiulcer properties.[116]

This supplement is available in chewable tablets and powdered form. The capsules may not be as effective as chewable tablets, as this supplement works best when mixed with saliva. This also allows it to have a direct effect on the stomach lining. The average dose for DGL is approximately one to three chewable tablets at a dose of 300-400 mg per tablet, about 20-30 minutes before each meal.

Slippery Elm

Slippery elm is a tree native to North America—specifically, the eastern region of Canada and the central and eastern regions of the United States. For centuries, Native Americans used the inner bark of this tree as an herbal remedy (for its demulcent and calming effects) to treat wounds, skin burns, and a number of internal diseases.

The benefits and medicinal properties of slippery elm bark are derived from the biochemical compounds that it contains. Some of these compounds are mucilage, tannins, fatty acids, and plant sterols.

The mucilage found in slippery elm bark is a type of soluble fiber that, when it comes in contact with water, forms a kind of thick gel that has a soothing and protective effect on the surfaces of irritated and inflamed tissues in the gastrointestinal tract. The tannins, fatty acids, and sterols found in the inner bark of this tree have been shown to have antioxidant and anti-inflammatory properties.

This supplement is available in capsules and powdered form. It is recommended that you choose its powdered form instead of the capsules, as the idea is to have the mucilages directly coat and protect your stomach lining. To prepare it, add one teaspoon of slippery elm powder to one cup of warm water and mix well for one minute before consuming it. (The mixture will thicken slightly.) It is also recommended that you take this remedy at least half an hour before eating and that you avoid taking it with other medications, as it can cause them to not be absorbed properly. Therefore, take it preferably two hours before or after you take any medication or supplement.

L-Glutamine

Glutamine, a non-essential amino acid that is found naturally in the body, is concentrated in large amounts in the muscles and is one of 20 amino acids involved in the composition of proteins that are responsible for maintaining cell health. This amino acid is considered non-essential because the body has the ability to synthesize, or produce by itself, enough quantities of it to meet its needs.

However, sometimes the body can increase the demand for glutamine, quickly leading to a depletion of the reserves of this amino acid (for example, when there is an increase in physical and mental stress or when someone suffers from trauma, burns, infections, or chronic and inflammatory diseases of the intestine). For this reason, in recent years, researchers have determined that this amino acid should be considered "conditionally essential" when you are critically ill or suffer from chronic diseases, as it is very important for healing processes and plays a fundamental role in the repair of damaged cells and tissues.[117] In this case, it helps repair the stomach lining.

Glutamine can be obtained naturally from high-protein foods such as chicken, red meat, fish, eggs, dairy products, and some vegetables. However, one of the main problems faced by people suffering from gastritis is that they often do not digest food well, which prevents them from making the most of all the nutrients. Often, this is due to the fact that the inflammation in the stomach does not allow digestion to be carried out correctly; nor is the secretion of gastric juices optimal. Also, the use of antacid medications does not enable optimal gastric acid secretion. This reduces the digestion and absorption of proteins, as stomach acid is necessary to denature them. This amino acid is the main fuel of the cells of the intestinal lining. When these cells receive the food that they love, the repair and regeneration of the intestinal walls is facilitated, which, in turn, prevents toxins and large molecules of undigested food from crossing the intestinal barrier and entering the bloodstream.[118]

This supplement is available in capsule and powdered form. It is recommended that you choose its powdered form, as the capsules do not contain over one gram of glutamine and, usually, the amount you will have to take exceeds that amount. While it is true that there is no specific dose for treating gastritis, many people have had good results taking between five and 10 grams daily (divided into several doses). My recommendation is that the dose be adjusted by a doctor familiar with this supplement (a naturopath or functional doctor).

The best way to take glutamine is to dilute the indicated amount in water at room temperature (never use hot water). Always take it away from meals and on an empty stomach so that it does not interact with other amino acids obtained from your diet.

Zinc Carnosine

Zinc carnosine is an artificially produced supplement composed of the mineral zinc and L-carnosine. When these two ingredients are bound together in a 1:1 ratio, they create a chelate compound that is much more effective and potent than each ingredient separately. In Japan, this supplement has been very popular since the mid-1990s as a treatment for gastric ulcers, dyspepsia, gastritis, and other digestive problems.[119]

By itself, zinc is very beneficial for digestive health in general. This mineral acts as an antioxidant and anti-inflammatory agent and is of vital importance to the immune system.[120] It is necessary for the production of stomach acid. Thus, a deficiency of this mineral can contribute to a lack of stomach acid.[121] Zinc deficiencies have also been associated with microbial infections, intestinal inflammation, late wound healing, and low immune system function.

On the other hand, L-carnosine, which is a dipeptide that is composed of the amino acids beta-alanine and L-histidine, has powerful antioxidant and healing properties. It helps transport the carnosine zinc complex to the site of inflammation or ulceration in the gastrointestinal tract, where the portions of L-carnosine and zinc can directly exert their healing and anti-inflammatory effects on the gastrointestinal tissue.[119]

This supplement is unique because, apart from stimulating the healing and repair of tissues in the gastrointestinal tract, it supports the natural mechanisms of stomach protection and helps stabilize the stomach and intestinal lining[122] without suppressing stomach acid or interfering with the normal digestive process. In addition, it has been shown that zinc carnosine inhibits the growth of Helicobacter pylori and the inflammatory response that causes it,[123] which increases its function as an antiulcer supplement. Unlike other forms of zinc, zinc carnosine causes fewer stomach problems, so it can be taken on an empty stomach as needed.

The most common dose used in clinical studies and that has produced better results is 150 mg of zinc carnosine (equivalent to 32 mg of zinc and 118 mg of L-carnosine) divided into two daily doses for eight weeks. However, although studies have shown that the optimal dose of zinc-carnosine is 150 mg per day, you can also choose to take 75 mg per day, as it has been shown that there is not much difference between the effects and final results obtained by taking any of the doses mentioned above.[119]

This supplement is available in capsules. You should take it between meals on an empty stomach or as directed by the manufacturer. If you experience stomach upset or any other symptoms when taking zinc-carnosine on an empty stomach, try taking it during a meal or after eating.

If taken at the recommended dose, zinc carnosine is safe and usually does not cause problems or side effects. However, overdosing of this supplement can cause zinc toxicity. It can also reduce copper levels in the body, which you should keep in mind when you are supplementing for a prolonged period of time, as you must maintain the balance of both minerals in the body. A good proportion of supplementation is that for every 15 mg of zinc, 1 mg of copper is needed.

Pregnant women, breastfeeding women, or people taking any prescription medication that can interact with zinc-carnosine should exercise caution. Therefore, it is always better to consult with a naturopath or functional doctor before you take this supplement.

Aloe Vera

Aloe vera is a plant that has been used for centuries due to its innumerable benefits and medicinal properties. In fact, there is evidence that it was used in ancient Egypt, where it was known as "the plant of immortality." While it is true that this plant contains a variety of vitamins, minerals, antioxidants, amino acids, enzymes, and secondary plant metabolites, what really makes it unique is a special compound known as acemannan—a mucilaginous polysaccharide that is present in aloe vera gel. This compound is known for its ability to strengthen the immune system and for its anti-inflammatory and antibacterial properties.[124]

However, the effectiveness of aloe vera is due not just to one or two compounds in particular; it is due to the synergistic action of all its active compounds. In itself, this plant is very beneficial for improving the health of the stomach when one is suffering from gastritis, as, apart from its anti-inflammatory effects, aloe vera gel helps regenerate the stomach lining and has a gastroprotective effect on the same.[125]

While you can prepare your own aloe vera remedy at home, you can also find it in the form of juice or concentrated powder, as well as consume it as a nutritional supplement.

Not every aloe vera product is recommended for those who suffer from gastritis. For example, aloe vera juice should be as pure as possible, preferably with a purity close to 99%, and should not contain acidulants such as citric acid, Vitamin C, or lemon. For this reason, it is important that you read the product label carefully so you will know that you are choosing a quality product that does not contain ingredients that will make your gastritis worse. The recommended amount of aloe vera juice to drink is a quarter to half a cup of juice, which is equivalent to two to four ounces, between or before meals. You can start by drinking a quarter cup and see if your stomach tolerates it, then increase the amount until you can drink half a cup of this juice.

If you can't find aloe vera juice, you can look for the powder concentrate. In itself, the powder concentrate is nothing more than dehydrated aloe vera gel. However, when choosing the powder concentrate, you must ensure that it comes only from the inner gel and not from the whole leaf, as the aloe vera outer leaf contains a substance called aloin, which can irritate the stomach lining and cause side effects such as diarrhea and abdominal pain. Another thing to keep in mind is that you should choose a powder concentrate that has been lyophilized or freeze-dried, as that way, the long-chain polysaccharides are better preserved. These are the components that give aloe vera some of its valuable and surprising medicinal properties.

If you get a good freeze-dried aloe vera supplement, I recommend that you add five grams (approximately two level teaspoons) of the powder concentrate to one liter of water. Then stir and let it dissolve completely (approximately 10 minutes). Once it has dissolved, place it in a refrigerator and consume it preferably within three to five days. You can start by drinking a third of a cup (80 ml) and then gradually increase the amount until you are drinking a cup and a quarter (300 ml) per day.

If you can't get pure juice or concentrated aloe vera powder, don't worry. Later, I'll show you how to prepare your own aloe vera remedy at home. And by the way, the internal use of aloe vera is contraindicated in pregnant or breastfeeding women and in young children.

Other Supplements

There are other supplements for gastritis that, while they do not have the gastroprotective, anti-inflammatory, and regenerative properties offered by the supplements mentioned above, can help improve digestion, increase nutrient absorption, and provide symptomatic relief of symptoms related to gastritis. However, while the following supplements can be of great help when one is suffering from gastritis, they are not absolutely essential to curing it.

Probiotics

The first supplements that I will talk about are probiotics, as many people do not know if they are really effective in treating gastritis. Probiotics themselves are nothing more than live bacteria considered to be "good" microorganisms that have proven beneficial for improving intestinal health. Probiotics contribute to the maintenance of balanced gut microbiota, which is important for the proper functioning of the digestive system.[126] They also help regulate the immune function of intestinal mucous cells and treat symptoms that may be related to gastritis, such as abdominal bloating, gas, stomach cramps, and acid reflux.

However, the problem with recommending probiotics is that no two people have the same gut microbiota—that is, the same community of living microorganisms that reside in the gastrointestinal tract. To determine which probiotic strains you need to take, you should go to a naturopath or functional doctor who has experience in the repopulation of gut microbiota. This way, the doctor can give you a complete stool test, see the state of your intestinal flora, and determine which microorganisms you already have.

If you decide to take probiotics on your own, you would be only guessing, as for a probiotic supplement to be effective, its formula must be adapted to the microbiota of the person. Therefore, when choosing a probiotic supplement, you should be particularly careful with those that have multiple strains and high CFUs (colony-forming units), as it is possible that your body will react to high amounts and new strains of bacteria in your intestine. Likely, trial and error is still the fastest way for you to get an answer.

My final observation regarding probiotics is, given that the microbiota in the intestine are as individual as a fingerprint, what works for one person may not work for you, and vice versa. That is why I recommend that you focus more on the stomach and not so much on the gut flora, as the latter will develop on their own as your stomach improves. In most cases, intestinal symptoms related to gastritis (e.g., abdominal bloating, gas, stomach cramps, etc.) are related to poorly digested food that passes into the intestine. Therefore, it doesn't matter how many probiotics you take; it is possible that they won't help you because that may not be the problem.

Digestive Enzymes

The second supplement that I will talk about is digestive enzymes. This supplement is often recommended for those suffering from gastritis. Digestive enzymes are substances that help break down (digest) food into tiny particles so that the body can absorb and take advantage of both the macronutrients (carbohydrates, fats, and proteins) and the micronutrients (vitamins and minerals) that foods contain.

The three main digestive enzymes are:

- **Protease** – an enzyme that breaks down proteins into amino acids.
- **Lipase** – an enzyme that breaks down fats into fatty acids.
- **Amylase** – an enzyme that breaks down carbohydrates, such as starches and sugar, into simple sugars and glucose.

A deficiency of these main enzymes can affect the absorption and utilization of the macronutrients and micronutrients in food. The presence of partially or poorly digested food can cause symptoms such as abdominal bloating, gas, stomach cramps, among others. Therefore, even if you have a proper diet, if your digestive system cannot transform and absorb nutrients properly, it will be much more difficult for the stomach to recover.

On the other hand, what happens in the stomach is that, when its lining is inflamed, less acid and fewer digestive enzymes are produced, which can cause digestion to become slow and heavy, leading you to experience symptoms of indigestion, stomach heaviness, and acid reflux. While it is true that proteases, lipases, and amylases are not produced in the stomach, but in the pancreas, if the chyme or bolus that leaves the stomach for the intestine is not acidic enough, the release of cholecystokinin (a hormone that stimulates the pancreas to release digestive enzymes in the duodenum) won't be proper.

As you can imagine, if that situation persists for a long time, it can have a negative downstream effect on the absorption and utilization of nutrients, leading to malnutrition or nutritional deficiencies.

With that in mind, you may be thinking that digestive enzyme supplementation is the most logical thing to do.

However, it is not a good idea to supplement with digestive enzymes if you do not know what is really happening inside your body. If you do not need them, you can cause your body to decrease its endogenous production of digestive enzymes. Therefore, to determine whether you are producing enough pancreatic enzymes, the best thing you can do is go to a naturopath or functional doctor so that he or she can test you for digestive enzyme deficiencies.

If you need to supplement with digestive enzymes, I recommend that you avoid those formulations that contain proteolytic enzymes such as protease, pepsin, and bromelain, as they can irritate your stomach lining and worsen some of the symptoms related to gastritis. However, if you do not find a digestive enzyme supplement without the proteolytic enzymes mentioned above, I recommend that you choose one that has the lowest protease concentration (preferably less than 20,000 HUT) and that you take it only with a protein-rich meal.

Other formulations that you should avoid are those that contain betaine HCL or betaine hydrochloride, which is nothing more than hydrochloric acid. If you have problems or a hard time digesting animal protein, you can try a papain supplement or eat a few pieces of papaya after consuming a protein-rich meal. Papaya is rich in papain, which is a proteolytic enzyme with anti-inflammatory properties that is not aggressive to the stomach.

Finally, my personal opinion regarding digestive enzyme supplements is that they are not at all necessary to heal your stomach, as all they do is help you digest food better. So, be careful when taking digestive enzymes. Take them only if necessary and do so under the supervision of a doctor.

Multivitamins

The last of the supplements I will talk about are multivitamins. When you suffer from gastritis, especially the chronic type, it is very common to develop vitamin and mineral deficiencies. The most common deficiencies are Vitamin B12 and iron, which can result in both pernicious anemia due to a lack of Vitamin B12 and iron deficiency anemia due to a lack of iron. However, in recent years, deficiencies of other vitamins and minerals, such as Vitamin D, folic acid, Vitamin C, and calcium, have been increasingly described in people suffering from gastritis.[127]

The first thing you should know about vitamins and minerals is that they are necessary for the body to function properly. Any deficiency of these can cause a number of symptoms and problems within your body.

Multivitamin supplements can provide the body with both the vitamins and minerals it needs, though eating a proper and balanced diet is still the best way to ensure good nutrition. Unfortunately, when one is suffering from gastritis, it is difficult to have a balanced diet and be able to properly absorb the nutrients that food contains. This is mainly due to the limitation or restriction that exists in the consumption of certain foods and to the problems of malabsorption related to low stomach acid.

Likewise, vitamin and mineral deficiencies, derived from a very strict diet or poor absorption of nutrients, can cause a number of symptoms that vary depending on the type of deficiency. Therefore, it is possible that many of the symptoms that you may be experiencing—such as fatigue or weakness, tiredness, sleepiness, dizziness, memory problems, mental confusion, and numbness or tingling in hands and legs—are due to vitamin and mineral deficiencies and not so much to symptoms directly related to inflammation in the stomach.

While it is true that taking a multivitamin can be beneficial when you are suffering from gastritis, there are several things you should keep in mind before you start doing so.

The first thing you should know is that it is much smarter to treat a deficiency of a specific mineral or vitamin than to take a multivitamin that contains high amounts of all vitamins and minerals. Therefore, my first recommendation is that you go to a doctor so that he or she can test you for vitamin and mineral deficiencies (or at least for Vitamin B12, folic acid, iron, and Vitamin D deficiencies).

The second thing to do is to be very careful when taking a multivitamin supplement in the form of tablets or capsules, as most of these supplements cause discomfort and stomach problems. This is primarily because multivitamin supplements often contain iron, zinc, and Vitamin C in forms that are very irritating to the stomach lining. Also, you should keep in mind that because many minerals and some vitamins are acid-dependent (that is, they require adequate levels of stomach acid to be absorbed), you may not absorb them well in the form of tablets or capsules. Therefore, my recommendation is that you choose this type of supplement in the form of a spray or sublingual drops, as in this way, they are better absorbed. Thus, you will avoid any discomfort in your stomach.

If you need to supplement with iron, consider taking it separately and, preferably, choose an iron supplement that is for people with a sensitive stomach, to avoid discomfort.

On the other hand, with so many brands and forms of minerals and vitamins, it is not possible to provide a definitive answer about which one you can or cannot take, as a specific brand or form could cause problems while another one does not.

It is also possible that you will not be able to find all the vitamins and minerals in the form of spray or sublingual drops. However, do not worry, as many vitamins and minerals are well absorbed in the form of capsules and tablets, since they do not require a very acidic pH to be absorbed. For example, magnesium in the form of glycinate has minimal gastrointestinal side effects, which are common with other forms of magnesium. I recommend only that you avoid most forms of iron and zinc (with the exception of zinc carnosine) and Vitamin C in the form of ascorbic acid.

Home Remedies for Gastritis

Potato Juice

The first of the home remedies I will talk about is the juice of raw potatoes, as it has been used for years to treat gastritis and gastric ulcers. Potatoes are especially rich in vitamins such as C, B3, B6, and B9, and minerals such as magnesium, phosphorus, and potassium. The alkaline properties of potato juice help it act as a natural antacid, thus calming stomach upset and relieving the pain of stomach ulcers.

Scientific research has shown that the gastroprotective effect of potato juice is due largely to the precipitate or sediment of the juice, which is composed mostly of starch. Meanwhile, the supernatant or the most liquid part of the juice is the one that confers the greatest antioxidant protection.[128]

Ingredients

• 1 or 2 large red or white potatoes

Preparation

1. Wash the potatoes well (they must be ripe), peel them, and remove all the black spots. Discard those that are green and that have many black spots (as they may have high amounts of a toxic substance called solanine).

2. Cut the potatoes into two halves and verify that they are not damaged inside. Then, place them in a juice extractor.

3. Take immediately to prevent the starch from precipitating at the bottom of the glass. It is preferable to take this juice once a day on an empty stomach.

Notes

• If you don't have a juice extractor, you can also use a blender. For this, just cut the potatoes into pieces, then blend them with half a cup of water and strain the mixture.

• If you do not like the taste of potato juice, you can mix it with carrot juice but do not add any sweeteners.

Chamomile Tea

Chamomile tea is one of the most popular teas to treat digestive problems. It is known mostly for its anti-inflammatory, soothing, and relaxing properties. Bisabolol, which is obtained from the essential oil of chamomile flower, is one of the active compounds that occur in greater concentration and is primarily responsible for the anti-inflammatory and regenerative effect of this herb on the stomach lining.[129]

Ingredients
- 1 tablespoon chamomile flowers (or one sachet)
- 1 cup of water
- Maple syrup to taste (optional)

Preparation
1. Bring the water to boil. When it starts boiling, turn off the heat.
2. Add chamomile flowers to boiled water. Cover with a lid and let stand for 15 minutes.
3. Strain and let it cool slightly. If you want to cool it faster, you can place the cup in a bowl filled with water. (Just make sure the water does not enter the cup containing the tea.)
4. Once the tea is warm or at room temperature, sweeten it to taste (optional). Take it about 20 or 30 minutes before eating.

Notes
- You can use this same recipe to prepare teas with other herbs and plants that have anti-inflammatory and soothing properties similar to chamomile, such as marshmallow root, fennel, ginger, lavender, and anise.
- It is important that you do not take this or any other tea when it is very hot. It is better to consume it warm or at room temperature.

Nopal Water

Nopal is a type of cactus native to America that has been shown to have excellent gastroprotective, antioxidant, and anti-inflammatory properties. The gastroprotective effects of nopal are attributed to the mucilages it contains inside its leaf. As we have mentioned before, this is a type of soluble fiber that provides a protective and regenerating effect on the stomach lining.[130] In addition, nopal is rich in polyphenols, a substance with antioxidant action that helps fight free radicals in the body.

Ingredients
- 1 nopal leaf
- 1 cup of water

Preparation
1. With a knife, remove all the thorns from the leaf and wash it well.
2. Cut the leaf into small pieces and place them along with the cup of water in a medium bowl. Cover it well and let it sit overnight to release the mucilages.
3. The next day, remove all the chopped pieces and drink the thick liquid 30 minutes before eating. It is recommended that you drink the nopal water about two or three times a day.

Note
- You can reuse the chopped pieces; you just have to add more water to the bowl or container to release more mucilages. However, keep in mind that the more times you reuse them, the lower their effectiveness will be, so I recommend that you reuse them only two or three times at most.

Aloe Vera

Aloe vera is a plant that, due to its anti-inflammatory, gastroprotective, and regenerative properties, has proved to be excellent for treating gastritis and its symptoms. Aloe vera is also rich in mucilage, which, as we mentioned above, has the ability to soothe and protect the stomach lining.

Ingredients

- 1 aloe vera leaf

Preparation

1. Cut a fifth of the aloe vera leaf (approximately a two-inch piece) and refrigerate the rest.
2. Then, cut the lateral rows of spines of the leaf and discard them. Rinse the leaf well.
3. Carefully remove the entire outer leaf. It is important that you remove it completely, as this part contains aloin, a bitter substance that can irritate the stomach lining.
4. Wash the aloe vera inner gel well and place it in a blender with a little water. Blend for about 30 seconds or until the mixture has a homogeneous consistency.
5. Take immediately or preferably 30 minutes before eating.

Notes

- Aloe vera is usually a little acidic (pH less than 5), so it is possible that some types of gastritis, especially the most severe cases, will not tolerate it well. If you can't tolerate it, try liquefying aloe vera gel with half a cup of papaya and a little water or plant-based milk.
- The internal use of aloe vera is contraindicated in pregnant or breastfeeding women and in young children.

CHAPTER 5:GETTING STARTED WITH THE MEAL PLAN

we have reached the third and last part of this book, in which we talk about the diet plan and recipes for gastritis. However, before we start, I would like you to know that the meal plan you will find in this part of the book has been designed specifically for those who prefer to follow a weekly meal plan without having to worry every day about what they are going to eat. In this way, you will know in advance what your next meal will be and that when you go to the supermarket, you can buy everything you will need to prepare your meals for the whole week.

However, it is not mandatory that you follow the specific meal plan that you will find later. If you prefer, you can create your own weekly meal plan with the recipes that I have included, or you can create your own recipes following the recommendations that I will give you next. In any case, it is recommended that you plan your meals in advance to avoid stressing or becoming anxious about not knowing what you are going to eat for your next meal or on the next day, and to make it easier for you to follow the diet described in this book.

The recipes that you will find later have been designed taking into account the irritating ingredients and some of the principles we have talked about throughout the healing program and in this book. Therefore, all the recipes you will find here are gastritis-friendly, as they were designed to cause as little damage or irritation as possible to the stomach lining of those suffering from gastritis. These were some of the criteria that were taken into account when I created each recipe:

Low acid (pH higher than 5)

Low fat (less than 10g per serving)

Low salt

No irritating ingredients

If you want to create your own recipes, I recommend that you take into account the criteria mentioned above and that you use the chart below to replace any irritating ingredient or condiment in a recipe that you want to prepare. Remember that the foods you use to create a recipe must come from the list of foods with a pH higher than 5 that we mentioned in the first step.

Gastritis-Friendly Ingredient Substitutions

REMOVE	REPLACE
Onion (raw or powder)	Fennel (bulb), leek (white part only), asafoetida
Garlic (raw or powder)	Asafoetida, ground cumin, Italian seasoning (without garlic) or a mixture of dried herbs (basil, oregano, rosemary, and thyme)
Chili powder, cayenne pepper,	Ground cumin, ground

paprika, black pepper	coriander
Vinegar, lime, lemon	Sumac (Turkish spice with a lemon-like taste) or grated zest of lemon, lime, or orange
Store-bought poultry seasoning	A mixture of salt with dried herbs (thyme, rosemary, basil, oregano, or others)
Chocolate	Carob (a great low-fat and caffeine-free substitute for chocolate)

NOTES

• Most of these substitutes should be used moderately and always for cooking (especially spices such as cumin and asafoetida). Dried herbs and sumac can be used uncooked. If you notice any reaction when you consume cumin or leek, replace them with another ingredient on the list. If you can't find asafoetida, sumac, or carob locally, you can get them online.

• In the last part of the recipes section, you will find some gastritis-friendly salad dressings, which you can use in your salads as a substitute for the salad dressings loaded with additives and irritating ingredients sold in supermarkets.

Tips for Creating Your Own Meal Plan

Before we start with the weekly meal plan, I would like to give you some tips and recommendations that will help you create your own diet plan.

- **Plan ahead.** Choose the meals or recipes that you will include in your weekly meal plan and write them down in your meal planner. Choose those recipes that sound attractive to you and that are easy to make. You can repeat a meal or recipe several times in the same week, although it is preferable that you eat as varied as possible. Do not forget to include snacks in your meal plan. Preferably, choose simple snacks that do not require much time for preparation.

- **Create your shopping list.** When you have your full weekly meal plan, create a shopping list with all the ingredients that you will need. This is a good way to avoid buying in excess and having to throw out expired or spoiled food. Once you have all the ingredients you will need, organize your shopping list based on where the items are located in the supermarket.

- **Cook for several days.** If you do not have much time to cook daily or if you simply do not want to be in the kitchen all day, I recommend that you take about two or three days a week to cook your meals and store them in the refrigerator in suitable containers (e.g. BPA-free plastic or glass food storage containers). The next day, or when you have to eat a specific meal, you just have to take it out of the refrigerator and heat it using the method you prefer. Cooking for several days will not only save you a lot of time but also help you avoid eating restaurant meals that may be prepared with irritating ingredients.

- **Change the menu regularly.** It is recommended that you change your meal menu on a regular basis to avoid eating always the same, which can also lead to nutritional deficiencies. Try to cook using new foods or add different recipes to your menu every week. This can be as simple as choosing different proteins for your salads each day or eating chicken with vegetables three nights a week, and fish or tofu with vegetables the other two. If you always choose boiled white rice, try changing it to sautéed potatoes or baked pumpkin. If you always eat broccoli, replace it with asparagus, Brussels sprouts, or other vegetables.

Now that you know what you can do to create your own meal plan, let's talk about everything you'll need to start with the weekly meal plan that I included.

Weekly Shopping List

The first thing we will talk about regarding the weekly meal plan is the shopping list, which has been included so that when you go to the supermarket, you will know in advance which foods, and how much, to buy so that you can make the respective recipes in the meal planner. Note that in the list you will see below, the ingredients listed as optional in the recipes and the ingredients for preparing the side dishes have not been included.

Therefore, I recommend that you take a look at each of the recipes that I have included in the meal planner and that you write down, on your weekly shopping list, the optional ingredients that you would like to add to the recipes. Do not forget to write down the ingredients of the side dishes (in the event that you want to prepare any of the dishes that I have included in Chapter 8) to accompany your main dishes.

Poultry and Eggs
- 3 boneless and skinless chicken breasts
- 6 ounces ground turkey breast
- 10 eggs

Fish
- 6 ounces salmon fillet
- 11 ounces cod fillet

Vegetables
- ¼ pound fresh spinach
- 1 pound broccoli
- ⅓ pound mushrooms
- ¼ pound Brussels sprouts
- ¾ pound pumpkin
- 5 medium carrots
- 1 small carrot
- 4 medium potatoes
- 1 small sweet potato
- 1 medium zucchini
- 1 fennel bulb
- 4 leeks
- 2 celery stalks
- 1 piece fresh ginger (about 1")
- 1 bunch fresh cilantro
- 1 bunch fresh parsley
- 1 bunch fresh basil
- 1 small packet fresh thyme

Fruits
- 6 ripe bananas
- ½ pound blueberries, strawberries, or mixed berries
- 4 ½ pounds of fresh fruits: watermelon, papaya, cantaloupe, Bosc pear, or dragon fruit
- 2 avocados

Bread and Grains

- 1 loaf gluten-free bread
- 1 small package gluten-free breadcrumbs (unseasoned)
- 1 small package gluten-free flour tortillas
- 1 package puffed rice cakes
- 1 package gluten-free pasta (preferably penne type)
- 1 package gluten-free pasta (rotini or fusilli type)
- 1 (5-ounce) package quick-cooking or unflavored instant oats

Others
- 4 liters unsweetened almond milk or other plant-based milk
- 1 (10-ounce) block extra-firm tofu
- 1 (8-ounce) package shelled walnuts

Kitchen Equipment and Pantry List

The following list details the essential items to store in your pantry and the kitchen equipment that you will need to prepare the recipes found in the meal planner. Most are affordable and easy to find. If, for some reason, you are unable to find the items locally, most are available online.

Pantry Items
- Extra virgin olive oil
- Sesame oil
- Sea salt or Himalayan pink salt
- Bragg liquid aminos or coconut aminos
- Maple syrup
- Almond butter
- Nutritional yeast
- Arrowroot flour or cornstarch
- Baking powder
- Ground oregano
- Dried oregano
- Ground cumin
- Dried thyme
- Dried rosemary

Essential Equipment
- Nonstick skillet
- 3 pots (small, medium, and large)
- 2 mixing bowls (small and medium)
- Potato masher
- Zester grater
- Spatula
- Balloon whisk
- Kitchen knives
- Complete set of measuring cups
- Complete set of measuring spoons
- Baking sheet

- Steamer basket
- Blender
- Small food processor

Tips for Meal Prep

If you do not have much time to cook daily or simply do not want to be in the kitchen all day, I recommend that you follow the next tips to prepare the meals found in the meal planner.

- Lunch and dinner meals can be prepared the previous night and stored in suitable containers (e.g. BPA-free plastic or glass food storage containers) so that you can heat them the next day or take them with you to work or wherever you go. Alternatively, you can take two or three days a week to prepare lunch and dinner for the next few days (up to three days maximum).
- Breakfast recipes are mostly easy to make and will not take you more than 15 minutes to prepare. Therefore, you do not need to prepare them the night before, except for the oatmeal, which you can prepare as indicated in the recipe and store in suitable containers—or you can add uncooked oats and plant-based milk to a glass jar and let it stand covered in the refrigerator overnight. The next day, you just have to add the other ingredients and enjoy your overnights oats.
- Fresh fruits for snacks can be chopped the day before and stored in the refrigerator in suitable containers, or you can chop enough fruits to store for up to three days (as long as you refrigerate and store them well in airtight containers). Toast can be prepared and stored in resealable bags to take with you wherever you go. You can prepare anti-inflammatory smoothies before you leave home and then store them in a thermal bottle to take with you.

Weekly Meal Plan

MONDAY

Breakfast	Scrambled Eggs with Spinach (see recipe)
Mid-morning	Chopped Fresh Fruits (see recipe)
Lunch	Chicken Vegetable Stir-Fry (see recipe)
Snack	Avocado Toast (see recipe)
Dinner	Creamy Mushroom Pasta (see recipe)

TUESDAY

Breakfast	Classic Oatmeal (see recipe)
Mid-morning	Toast or Rice Cake with Almond Butter (see recipe)
Lunch	Creamy Pumpkin Soup (see recipe)
Snack	Anti-Inflammatory Smoothie (see recipe)
Dinner	Baked Cod with Brussels Sprouts (see recipe)

WEDNESDAY

Breakfast	Banana Oat Smoothie (see recipe)
Mid-morning	Toast or Rice Cake with Almond Butter (see recipe)
Lunch	Grilled Chicken with Spinach and Mushrooms (see recipe)
Snack	Chopped Fresh Fruits (see recipe)
Dinner	Cream of Broccoli Soup with Toast (see recipe)

THURSDAY

Breakfast	Scrambled Eggs with Spinach (see recipe)
Mid-morning	Chopped Fresh Fruits (see recipe)
Lunch	Veggie Tofu Stir-Fry (see recipe)
Snack	Toast or Rice Cake with Almond Butter (see recipe)
Dinner	Chicken Vegetable Soup (see recipe)

FRIDAY

Breakfast	Classic Oatmeal (see recipe)
Mid-morning	Avocado Toast (see recipe)
Lunch	Baked Turkey Meatballs (see recipe)

Snack	Anti-Inflammatory Smoothie (see recipe)
Dinner	Roasted Vegetable Burrito (see recipe)
SATURDAY	
Breakfast	Banana Berry Smoothie (see recipe)
Mid-morning	Toast or Rice Cake with Almond Butter (see recipe)
Lunch	Pesto Pasta with Tofu (see recipe)
Snack	Chopped Fresh Fruits (see recipe)
Dinner	Baked Chicken Tenders (see recipe)
SUNDAY	
Breakfast	Banana Oat Pancakes (see recipe)
Mid-morning	Chopped Fresh Fruits (see recipe)
Lunch	Glazed Salmon with Broccoli (see recipe)
Snack	Toast or Rice Cake with Almond Butter (see recipe)
Dinner	Fish Stew (see recipe)

Thoughts on the Meal Plan and Recipes

Before you go on to the recipes and start following the weekly meal plan you just saw, I would like to clarify some things about the recipes and this meal plan.

Most of the recipes for lunch and dinner are accompanied only by vegetables. If you want to accompany them with a side dish, you can choose any of those in Chapter 8 or another recipe you have in mind and that is not in this book. However, if you choose a recipe that is not in this book, it should be gastritis-friendly so that you avoid irritating your stomach lining. Also, do not overdo it with the portions of the side dishes, as you want to avoid delaying digestion too much by mixing a lot of carbohydrates with proteins. As a general rule, the amount of carbohydrates you add to a protein-rich meal should not exceed one cup.

Many of the recipes you will see below, especially those for lunch and dinner, are mostly one or two servings—that is, for one or two people. Keep this in mind when preparing a recipe, as it is possible that you will be able to eat only one serving and that the other portion will have to be stored in the refrigerator or shared with someone else. If you want to share a one-serving recipe with one or more people, do not forget to double or multiply the ingredients of the recipe so that everyone can eat.

If you experience an increase in symptoms after you start to follow the meal plan, this may be because you are unable to tolerate some new foods. The most common intolerances are egg, oatmeal, bananas, and other foods that you will find in the recipes. If you suspect that there is a particular food that you do not tolerate, remove it for a week or two and then reintroduce it.

In most cases, intolerances are related to intestinal problems, the severity of gastritis, and poor gastroprotection. If this is your case, it is recommended that you protect your stomach as much as possible and that you increase gastroprotection naturally by consuming linoleic-acid-rich foods. This will increase the production of prostaglandins in the stomach. Do not forget to treat any other intestinal problems that may be causing you food intolerances.

CHAPTER 6:BREAKFAST RECIPES

Classic Oatmeal

This comforting, warm, and creamy porridge is an excellent way to start the day. Oatmeal provides vitamins and minerals, and, being rich in soluble fiber, contributes to a healthy digestive system.

Servings: 1 | **Preparation:** 5 minutes | **Cooking:** 10 minutes

Ingredients

½ cup quick-cooking or unflavored instant oats

1 cup unsweetened almond milk or other plant-based milk

1 ripe banana, sliced

A pinch of salt

¼ teaspoon vanilla extract (optional)

1 tablespoon coconut flakes or chopped walnuts (optional)

1 tablespoon maple syrup (optional, to drizzle on top)

Preparation

1.   In a small saucepan over medium-high heat, add the milk, oats, pinch of salt, and vanilla (if using). Cook, stirring for about 5 minutes or until it starts to boil.

2.   Once it starts to boil, reduce the heat to low and cook, stirring constantly, for about 5 minutes or until it begins to thicken.

3.   Remove from heat and pour it in a bowl. Serve with banana slices, coconut flakes, or walnuts and maple syrup on top (if using these optional ingredients).

Notes

•   If you don't tolerate oatmeal, you can try the rice porridge recipe (see recipe) that I included later.

•   You can substitute the banana for half a ripe Bosc pear, sliced and peeled, or another type of fruit that has a pH greater than 5.

Per serving: (1 bowl) Calories: 295; Total fat: 5.7g; Protein: 8g; Carbohydrates: 48.6g; Fiber: 7.2g

Scrambled Eggs with Spinach

These tasty scrambled eggs with spinach are ideal for breakfast, as they are easy to prepare and give your body the proteins it needs to start the day.

Servings: 1 | **Preparation:** 10 minutes | **Cooking:** 5 minutes

Ingredients

1 large egg
2 egg whites
1 cup fresh spinach, chopped
½ teaspoon olive or coconut oil
¼ teaspoon salt
1 tablespoon black olives, chopped (optional)
1 slice gluten-free toast or another side dish

Preparation

1.   In a medium bowl, beat the egg, egg whites, and salt. Add spinach and black olives (if using). Mix all the ingredients well.
2.   Heat a nonstick skillet over medium heat and cover with olive oil. Pour the egg mixture into the pan and cook, stirring constantly, for about 2 minutes or until the egg and spinach are cooked.
3.   Remove from heat and transfer to a plate. Serve with the slice of bread or another side dish (a small or medium potato or sweet potato, cooked and skinless).

Note

•   You can substitute spinach for kale. On the other hand, if you do not tolerate eggs, try the vegetarian recipe (<u>see recipe</u>) that I included later, which is very similar to this but, instead of eggs, has tofu.

Per serving: (3 eggs scrambled with a slice of toast) Calories: 210; Total fat: 9g; Protein: 15g; Carbohydrates: 15g; Fiber: 1.2g

Banana Oat Pancakes

These simple and healthy pancakes are an excellent alternative to traditional pancakes, as they are made with oats instead of wheat flour and do not require eggs or dairy for their preparation.

Servings: 1 | **Preparation:** 10 minutes | **Cooking:** 15 minutes

Ingredients

½ cup quick-cooking oats or oat flour
½ medium ripe banana
¼ cup unsweetened almond milk or other plant-based milk
1 teaspoon baking powder
A pinch of salt
½ teaspoon vanilla extract (optional)
1 tablespoon maple syrup (to drizzle on top)

Preparation

1.   If using quick-cooking oats, add them to the blender and pulse until they are well-ground. Otherwise (if using oat flour), add all the ingredients (except maple syrup) and blend until the mixture is smooth. Pour the mixture into a medium bowl and set aside.
2.   Heat a nonstick skillet over medium heat. Pour ¼ cup of the mixture into the prepared pan and cook until small bubbles form in the center of the pancakes or until the bottom is golden-brown, about 1 or 2 minutes. Turn with a spatula and cook for 1 or 2 minutes on the other side. Repeat with the remaining mixture.
3.   Serve with maple syrup and half a ripe banana sliced on top.

Note

•   If you do not tolerate these pancakes, try the other pancake recipe (see recipe) that I included later.

Per serving: (2 ½ pancakes) Calories: 272; Total fat: 5.6g; Protein: 8.6g; Carbohydrates: 43g; Fiber: 4.9g

Rice Porridge

A very rich and great alternative to porridge. Perfect for those who can't eat or tolerate oatmeal.

Servings: 1 | **Preparation:** 5 minutes | **Cooking:** 10 minutes

Ingredients

1 cup cooked white rice
1 cup unsweetened almond milk or other plant-based milk
1 ripe banana, sliced
1 or 2 tablespoons maple syrup
½ teaspoon vanilla extract (optional)
1 tablespoon coconut flakes or chopped walnuts (optional)
1 tablespoon maple syrup (optional, to drizzle on top)

Preparation

1.   In a medium saucepan, add the cooked rice, milk, maple syrup, and vanilla (if using) and let it boil.
2.   Once it starts to boil, reduce the heat to low and cook, stirring constantly, for about 5-10 minutes, until it absorbs part of the liquid and begins to thicken.
3.   Remove from heat and pour it into a bowl. Serve with banana slices, coconut flakes, or walnuts and maple syrup on top (if using these optional ingredients).

Notes

•   The rice to be used in this recipe must be previously cooked without oil and without salt.
•   You can substitute the banana for half a ripe Bosc pear, sliced and peeled, or another type of fruit that has a pH greater than 5.

Per serving: (1 bowl) Calories: 398; Total fat: 3.5g; Protein: 7g; Carbohydrates: 82g; Fiber: 3.6g

Tofu Scramble

This scrambled tofu is an excellent vegetarian alternative to the typical scrambled eggs. Tofu is a protein-rich food that contains all the essential amino acids that your body needs.

Servings: 2 | **Preparation:** 10 minutes | **Cooking:** 10 minutes

Ingredients

6 ounces (170g) firm tofu, drained
1 cup fresh spinach, chopped
¼ teaspoon ground turmeric (to add color)
¼ teaspoon ground cumin
1 or 2 tablespoons nutritional yeast (optional)
¼ teaspoon salt
½ teaspoon olive or coconut oil
1 slice gluten-free toast or another side dish

Preparation

1.   Place the tofu in a medium bowl and crush it with a potato masher or fork (or with your clean hands) until you get a texture similar to that of scrambled eggs. Add the other ingredients (except spinach and oil) and mix well.
2.   Heat a pan over high heat and cover with olive oil. Add the tofu and cook, stirring constantly, for about 3 or 5 minutes, or until the water from the tofu evaporates.
3.   Add the spinach and cook, stirring constantly, for another 5 minutes or until spinach is wilted.
4.   Serve with the slice of bread or another side dish (a small or medium-sized potato or sweet potato, cooked and skinless).

Note

•   Turmeric and cumin are two very unpredictable spices, as they cause stomach discomfort in some people. Therefore, it is recommended that you try the recipe and see how well you tolerate it.

Per serving: (3 ounces of tofu scrambled without toast) Calories: 119; Total fat: 7.2g; Protein: 13.3g; Carbohydrates: 1.7g; Fiber: 1.4g

3-Ingredient Pancakes

These fluffy and naturally sweet pancakes are really easy to make—and, best of all, they require only 3 ingredients for their preparation! They are ideal for a quick breakfast or lazy weekend mornings.

Servings: 1 | **Preparation:** 5 minutes | **Cooking:** 5-10 minutes

Ingredients

1 very ripe banana

1 large egg

¼ cup gluten-free all-purpose flour (see notes)

Preparation

1.   In a medium bowl, mash the banana well with a fork. Add the egg and mix well.
2.   Combine the gluten-free flour with the wet ingredients. (Be sure to break up lumps that have formed.)
3.   Heat a nonstick skillet over medium heat. Pour ¼ cup of the mixture into the prepared pan and cook until small bubbles form in the center or until the pancakes are golden-brown on the bottom, about 1 or 2 minutes. Turn with a spatula and cook for 1 or 2 minutes on the other side. Repeat with the remaining mixture.
4.   Serve with maple syrup and half a ripe banana sliced on top (optional).

Notes

•   If you want the pancakes to be fluffier, you can add ½ teaspoon of baking powder to the mixture.
•   If you can't find gluten-free all-purpose flour, use oat flour or gluten-free pancake mix.

Per serving: (3 pancakes) Calories: 283; Total fat: 6.3g; Protein: 10.6g; Carbohydrates: 43.9g; Fiber: 5.6g

Mushroom and Spinach Omelette

A rich and tasty omelette loaded with nutritious vegetables such as spinach, mushrooms, and zucchini. Ideal for when you need a simple but nutritious breakfast.

Servings: 1 | **Preparation:** 10 minutes | **Cooking:** 10 minutes

Ingredients

1 large egg
2 egg whites
½ cup fresh mushrooms, sliced
1 cup fresh spinach
½ cup zucchini, sliced (optional)
1 teaspoon olive or coconut oil
¼ teaspoon salt
1 slice gluten-free toast or another side dish

Preparation

1.   In a small bowl, beat the egg, egg whites, and salt. Set aside.
2.   In a nonstick skillet, heat the oil over medium-high heat. Add the mushrooms and zucchini (if using) and cook, stirring frequently, for about 3 or 5 minutes, or until the vegetables are tender.
3.   Add the spinach and cook, stirring until it wilts. Set aside and reduce heat to medium.
4.   Pour the eggs into the pan (or in another lightly greased nonstick skillet). As the eggs are cooked, lift the edges and slightly tilt the pan to cover the sides and allow the raw part to flow underneath.
5.   When the eggs are cooked, place the mushrooms, spinach, and zucchini (if using) in the center of the tortilla. If desired, sprinkle with a little salt on top. Gently fold the tortilla in half and transfer to a plate.
6.   Serve with the slice of bread or another side dish (a small or medium potato or sweet potato, cooked and skinless).

Per serving: (1 omelette) Calories: 227; Total fat: 9.8g; Protein: 17g; Carbohydrates: 15.4g; Fiber: 1.6g

Banana Berry Smoothie

A rich banana and berry smoothie that, apart from being healthy and easy to prepare, provides your body with antioxidants and good fats from berries and almond butter.

Servings: 1 | **Preparation:** 5 minutes | **Cooking:** N/A

Ingredients

1 very ripe banana

½ cup blueberries, strawberries, or mixed berries

1 cup unsweetened almond milk or other plant-based milk

½ tablespoon almond butter

1 or 2 tablespoons pea or hemp protein (optional)

Preparation

1.   Place all the ingredients in a blender and pulse for a minute or until the mixture has a smooth consistency.

2.   Serve immediately and enjoy.

Notes

•   If you desire, you can substitute almond butter for a tablespoon of walnuts or shelled hemp seeds.

•   It is advisable to freeze the bananas and/or berries beforehand to avoid adding ice to the smoothie.

Per serving: (2 cups approx.) Calories: 248; Total fat: 8g; Protein: 4.8g; Carbohydrates: 36g; Fiber: 6g

Banana Oat Smoothie

This delicious banana oat smoothie is ideal for those lazy mornings or when you need a quick but satisfying breakfast.

Servings: 1 | **Preparation:** 5 minutes | **Cooking:** N/A

Ingredients

1 very ripe banana
¼ cup rolled or quick-cooking oats
1 cup unsweetened almond milk or other plant-based milk
½ tablespoon almond butter
1 tablespoon carob powder (optional, but recommended)

Preparation

1.   Place the oats in the blender and pulse until well ground. Add the other ingredients and pulse for a minute or until the mixture gets a smooth consistency.
2.   Serve immediately and enjoy.

Notes

•   If you desire, you can substitute almond butter for a tablespoon of walnuts or shelled hemp seeds.
•   It is recommended that you soak the oats in water overnight, as this way they will be easier to digest. The next day, you just have to strain the oats and add them to the smoothie.

Per serving: (2 cups approx.) Calories: 266; Total fat: 8.7g; Protein: 7g; Carbohydrates: 37g; Fiber: 5.9g

Avocado Toast with Egg

This simple and tasty recipe is really easy to make and requires few ingredients. It is ideal for a quick and light breakfast or snack.

Servings: 1 | **Preparation:** 5 minutes | **Cooking:** N/A

Ingredients

⅓ cup avocado, peeled and diced

1 tablespoon fresh cilantro, finely chopped

1 cooked large egg, sliced

Salt to taste

2 slices gluten-free toast

Preparation

1.   In a small bowl, add the avocado and mash it using a potato masher or fork. Add the cilantro and salt to taste and mix well.

2.   Pour the avocado mixture over the toast and place the egg slices on top. Serve and enjoy.

Notes

•   Depending on your tolerance, you can add more avocado to toast.

•   On the other hand, if you want to add more protein, you can add 1 or 2 chopped cooked egg whites or ⅓ cup of scrambled tofu on top of the avocado.

Per serving: (two slices of toast) Calories: 205; Total fat: 9.7g; Protein: 4.5g; Carbohydrates: 28g; Fiber: 5.3g

CHAPTER 7:LUNCH AND DINNER RECIPES

Chicken Vegetable Stir-Fry

This tasty Chinese-style stir-fry is loaded with nutritious vegetables and topped with a delicious and healthy homemade stir-fry sauce. It's a perfect accompaniment to white rice or cauliflower rice.

Servings: 1 | **Preparation:** 20 minutes | **Cooking:** 15 minutes

Ingredients

½ boneless, skinless chicken breast, cut into pieces
¾ cup broccoli florets, cut into pieces
½ medium carrot, peeled and julienned
¼ medium zucchini, sliced
⅓ cup mushrooms, sliced (optional)
½ tablespoon of olive or coconut oil
½ teaspoon ginger, grated
1 ½ tablespoons coconut aminos or Bragg liquid aminos
2 teaspoons sesame oil
½ teaspoon arrowroot flour or cornstarch (see notes)

Preparation

1.   In a nonstick skillet or wok over medium-high heat, add the oil, ginger, and chicken. Cook, stirring occasionally, until the chicken is cooked or slightly browned. Remove the chicken from the pan and set it aside.
2.   Add the vegetables to the pan and cook, stirring frequently, until tender, about 5 to 7 minutes.
3.   In a small bowl, mix the coconut aminos or Bragg liquid aminos, sesame oil, and arrowroot flour or cornstarch.
4.   Add the chicken back to the pan and pour the stir-fry sauce on top. Stir well and simmer, stirring occasionally, for an additional 2 or 3 minutes. Serve and enjoy.

Note

•   If you use cornstarch instead of arrowroot flour, I recommend that you use one that is NON-GMO (non-transgenic).

Per serving: (2 ½ cups approx.) Calories: 179; Total fat: 6.6g; Protein: 21.4g; Carbohydrates: 6g; Fiber: 6.3g

Grilled Chicken with Spinach and Mushrooms

This exquisite recipe for grilled chicken breast over a spinach and mushroom bed is not only tasty but also simple. It provides your body with a large amount of protein and amino acids.

Servings: 1 | **Preparation:** 15 minutes | **Cooking:** 15 minutes

Ingredients

1 boneless, skinless chicken breast
1 cup fresh spinach
2 or 3 medium mushrooms, sliced
¼ leek (white part only), finely chopped
2 teaspoons olive oil, divided
¼ teaspoon salt
½ teaspoon dried oregano

Preparation

1.   In a medium bowl, combine the salt, oregano, and a teaspoon of olive oil. Add the chicken and cover generously with the mixture. Let stand for 20-30 minutes.
2.   Heat a grill pan or nonstick skillet over medium heat and cook the chicken for about 5-7 minutes. Turn on the other side and cook for another 5-7 minutes or until the chicken is cooked. Set aside.
3.   In a nonstick skillet over medium heat (you can use the same pan), add the remaining oil and the chopped leek and cook, stirring constantly, for about 2 or 3 minutes or until the leek is a little browned.
4.   Add the mushrooms to the pan and cook for 2 or 3 more minutes or until tender. Finally, add spinach and cook until it wilts. Place the mushrooms and spinach on a plate and serve with the chicken on top of the vegetables.

Note

•   If you desire, instead of sautéing the mushrooms, you can prepare a mushroom sauce (see recipe) to pour over the chicken breast.

Per serving: (1 chicken breast approx.) Calories: 234; Total fat: 6g; Protein: 40g; Carbohydrates: 0g; Fiber: 0g

Baked Cod with Brussels Sprouts

A simple and healthy recipe for baked cod covered with aromatic herbs that, apart from having an exquisite flavor, is easy to make and requires few ingredients.

Servings: 1 | **Preparation:** 20 minutes | **Cooking:** 20 minutes

Ingredients

5-ounce cod fillet

1 teaspoon dried or fresh herbs (thyme, rosemary, parsley, or sage)

2 teaspoons olive oil, divided

¼ teaspoon salt

¼ pound Brussels sprouts (1 ¼ cups approx.) (see notes)

Preparation

1.   Preheat the oven to 375°F. Grease a baking sheet with nonstick spray oil (or cover with parchment paper). Set aside.
2.   In a small bowl, mix a teaspoon of olive oil, salt, and dried or fresh herbs.
3.   Place the cod fillet on the prepared baking sheet and distribute the herb mixture with oil evenly over the cod.
4.   Trim the ends of the Brussels sprouts and cut them in half through the root. Place the cut cabbages in a medium bowl. Pour over the remaining teaspoon of olive oil and sprinkle with salt to taste. Mix well.
5.   Distribute the Brussels sprouts on the prepared baking sheet together with the cod and bake for 12-15 minutes or until the fish crumbles easily with a fork.
6.   After the first 12-15 minutes, remove the cod from the oven and bake the Brussels sprouts for another 10-15 minutes or until tender and golden-brown.
7.   Transfer the Brussels sprouts to a plate and serve with the baked cod.

Notes

•   Brussels sprouts can be replaced by spinach, broccoli, or steamed asparagus, or any other vegetable you want to use as a side dish.
•   On the other hand, if you can't find cod, replace it with tilapia or salmon.

Per serving: (5 ounces of cod) Calories: 189; Total fat: 1g; Protein: 32g; Carbohydrates: 0g; Fiber: 0g

Chicken Vegetable Soup

This comforting and soothing chicken soup loaded with nutritious vegetables is perfect for a light dinner in the middle of the week or for when you're in the middle of a flare-up and you need something light for your stomach.

Servings: 4 | **Preparation:** 15 minutes | **Cooking:** 30 minutes

Ingredients

1 boneless, skinless chicken breast, cut into pieces
2 celery stalks, chopped
1 medium carrot, peeled and sliced
1 or 2 medium potatoes, cut into pieces
1 leek (white and light green parts only), washed and chopped
1 cup pumpkin, peeled and diced
6 cups water or vegetable broth (see recipe)
1 tablespoon extra virgin olive oil
2 or 3 teaspoons salt
4 sprigs fresh thyme (or 1 teaspoon dried thyme)
½ teaspoon ground coriander (optional)

Preparation

1.   In a large pot, heat the oil over medium heat and gently sauté the leek and chicken for about 5 minutes or until the leek is tender and the chicken begins to lose its pinkish color.

2.   Add the chopped vegetables, water or vegetable broth, 2 teaspoons salt, thyme, and coriander (if using) and bring to a boil.

3.   Once it starts to boil, reduce the heat to low and cover the pot with a lid. Let the soup simmer until the chicken is well cooked and the vegetables are tender, 25 to 30 minutes.

4.   Taste the soup and, if necessary, add 1 more teaspoon of salt. Serve warm and enjoy.

Per serving: (1 medium bowl) Calories: 149; Total fat: 4.9g; Protein: 11g; Carbohydrates: 12.6g; Fiber: 2.5g

Baked Turkey Meatballs

These tasty baked turkey meatballs are a healthy alternative to traditional beef-based meatballs. They're perfect to serve with zucchini noodles or you can cover them with a rich mushroom sauce.

Servings: 2 | **Preparation:** 10 minutes | **Cooking:** 20 minutes

Ingredients

6 ounces ground turkey breast (or ground chicken)
½ cup gluten-free breadcrumbs
1 large egg, beaten
2 tablespoons fresh parsley, chopped
2 tablespoons leek (white part only), finely chopped
½ teaspoon ground oregano
¼ teaspoon ground cumin
½ teaspoon salt

Preparation

1.   Preheat the oven to 375°F. Cover a baking sheet with parchment paper or lightly grease it with nonstick spray oil. Set aside.
2.   In a medium bowl, add the ground turkey, breadcrumbs, egg, salt, parsley, leek, cumin, and oregano and mix well. (You can do this with your hands.)
3.   Form about 10 or 12 balls with your hands and place them on the prepared baking sheet.
4.   Bake for about 15-20 minutes or until the meatballs are cooked. Serve and enjoy.

Note

•   If you desire, you can prepare the mushroom sauce (see recipe) that I included in the chapter containing extra recipes and then pour this sauce over your meatballs.

Per serving: (6 meatballs) Calories: 285; Total fat: 8g; Protein: 31g; Carbohydrates: 18g; Fiber: 1.9g

Glazed Salmon with Broccoli

A rich and tasty salmon covered with a sweet-salty glaze that, apart from giving the salmon an exquisite flavor, creates a delicious caramelized crust.

Servings: 2 | **Preparation:** 10 minutes | **Cooking:** 20 minutes

Ingredients

5-ounce salmon fillet
3 tablespoons maple syrup or honey
2 tablespoons of Bragg liquid aminos or coconut aminos
1 teaspoon miso paste (optional)
1 teaspoon ginger, grated
1 cup broccoli florets, rinsed

Preparation

1.   In a medium bowl, mix Bragg liquid aminos or coconut aminos, maple or honey syrup, ginger, and miso (if using). Reserve about 2 tablespoons of the glaze to pour over the salmon at the end.
2.   Place the salmon in the mixture and let it marinate at room temperature for 15 minutes (or up to 30 minutes in the refrigerator) before cooking. Be sure to cover the salmon well with the marinade.
3.   While the salmon is marinating, fill a medium pot with about 1 inch of water. Place a steamer basket inside the pot (it should not touch the water) and bring to a boil.
4.   Place the broccoli in the steamer basket and cover with a lid. Let the broccoli steam for about 4 to 5 minutes or until it softens a little. Remove the broccoli from the pot and transfer it onto a plate. Season with salt and set aside.

IF BAKING

1.   Preheat the oven to 400°F. and grease a baking sheet with oil (preferably nonstick spray oil).
2.   Place the salmon on the prepared baking sheet and bake for about 15 minutes or until the salmon crumbles easily with a fork.
3.   Roast for 1 to 2 minutes or until the top of the salmon is lightly browned. Watch closely so that it does not burn.
4.   Remove from the oven and, if desired, drizzle or brush the salmon with a little of the remaining marinade. Let it stand a few minutes before serving with broccoli.

IF GRILLING

1.   Preheat a grill pan over medium heat and lightly grease it.
2.   Place the salmon on the greased grill pan and cook for 4 to 6 minutes. Turn and cook on the other side for approximately 3-4 minutes or until the salmon crumbles easily with a fork. (The salmon should still be a little pink in the middle.)
3.   Remove from the grill and, if desired, drizzle or brush the salmon with a little of the remaining marinade. Let stand for a few minutes before serving with broccoli.

Per serving: (2.5 ounces of salmon, 1 cup of broccoli) Calories: 184; Total fat: 6g; Protein: 18g; Carbohydrates: 6g; Fiber: 5g

Baked Chicken Tenders

These crispy baked chicken tenders are a tasty and healthy alternative to fried chicken tenders. They're an ideal accompaniment to a cup of steamed vegetables and/or mashed potatoes.

Servings: 1 | **Preparation:** 10 minutes | **Cooking:** 20 minutes

Ingredients

1 large egg
½ boneless, skinless chicken breast, cut into six strips
¼ cup gluten-free breadcrumbs
½ teaspoon dried thyme
1 teaspoon dried oregano
½ teaspoon salt

Preparation

1.   Preheat the oven to 425°F. Cover a baking sheet with parchment paper or grease it with nonstick spray oil. Set aside.
2.   In a medium bowl, add the breadcrumbs, thyme, oregano, and salt. Mix well.
3.   Beat the egg in another small bowl. Dip the chicken strips in the beaten egg and then in the breadcrumb mixture. Shake any excess coating off the strips.
4.   Place the chicken strips on the prepared baking sheet and bake for 15 to 20 minutes, turning once, until the chicken strips are lightly browned.
5.   Serve with cooked vegetables or the side dish of your choice.

Note

•   You can use this same recipe to make turkey or fish tenders. Just replace the chicken with an equal amount of skinless turkey breast or fish of your choice.

Per serving: (3 chicken strips) Calories: 247; Total fat: 8.4g; Protein: 30g; Carbohydrates: 9.5g; Fiber: 1g

Fish Stew

This hearty and flavorful fish stew makes a great midweek meal to warm you up in on a cold winter evening. It's a versatile recipe and you can use whatever white fish you like for your perfect fish stew.

Servings: 2 | **Preparation:** 10 minutes | **Cooking:** 20 minutes

Ingredients

1 leek (white part only), washed and chopped

6 ounces cod or halibut, skin removed and cut into bite-size pieces

1 fennel bulb, cored and chopped

1-2 tablespoons fennel fronds or fresh parsley, chopped

2 carrots, peeled and diced

1 medium potato, peeled and quartered

1 tablespoon olive oil

3 cups vegetable broth (see recipe)

1 teaspoon arrowroot flour or NON-GMO cornstarch

½ teaspoon salt

Preparation

1. Heat the oil in a large pot over medium-high heat. Add the fennel and leek, and sauté for about 5 minutes, or until the vegetables start to brown.

2. Add the fish and cook, stirring frequently, for about 3-4 minutes.

3. In a medium bowl, mix the arrowroot flour or cornstarch with the broth. Then add it to the pot, along with the carrots, potato, and salt.

4. Cook, stirring occassionally, until the potato and carrots are soft and tender, about 15 minutes.

5. Stir in the fennel fronds or fresh parsley just before serving. Serve warm and enjoy!

Per serving: (2 cups approx.) Calories: 298; Total fat: 8g; Protein: 23g; Carbohydrates: 26g; Fiber: 8g

Cream of Broccoli Soup

This classic and delicious cream of broccoli soup is super-healthy and very nutritious. Best of all, it does not require cream or butter for its creamy texture.

Servings: 2 | **Preparation:** 15 minutes | **Cooking:** 20 minutes

Ingredients

2 cups broccoli florets, rinsed
2 cups water or vegetable broth (see recipe)
½ cup unsweetened almond milk or other plant-based milk
½ cup leek (white part only), washed and finely chopped
1 medium potato, peeled and cut into pieces
1 teaspoon olive or coconut oil
1 teaspoon salt

Preparation

1.   In a medium saucepan, heat the oil over medium-high heat. Add the chopped leek and cook, stirring constantly, until tender, about 5 minutes.
2.   Add the broccoli, potato, vegetable broth, and salt. Bring to a boil.
3.   Once it starts to boil, reduce the heat to medium and cook for 15 minutes or until the vegetables are soft.
4.   Remove from heat and allow the soup to cool slightly. Then transfer it to a blender and add the milk. Blend until it has a smooth consistency.
5.   Place the mixture in the pot again over medium heat and cook for an additional 2 or 3 minutes or until the soup thickens slightly.
6.   Serve warm with slices of toast (optional).

Per serving: (1 medium bowl) Calories: 131; Total fat: 2.2g; Protein: 5g; Carbs: 20g; Fiber: 4.3g

Creamy Pumpkin Soup

A comforting, rich, and creamy pumpkin soup full of flavor and prepared without any cream. Perfect for those cold winter days and ideal to accompany with slices of crusty toast.

Servings: 1 | **Preparation:** 15 minutes | **Cooking:** 25 minutes

Ingredients

1 ¼ cups (150g approx.) pumpkin, peeled, seeded, and diced

½ medium carrot, peeled and sliced

½ medium potato, peeled and cut into pieces

½ leek (white part only), washed and sliced

1 cup water or vegetable broth (see recipe)

½ tablespoon olive oil

½ teaspoon salt

¼ teaspoon ground coriander (optional)

Preparation

1.   In a medium saucepan over medium heat, add the oil and chopped vegetables and cook, stirring occasionally, for about 5 minutes. Add water or vegetable broth and bring to a boil.

2.   When it starts to boil, add salt and ground coriander (if using). Let the vegetables cook over medium-high heat for about 15 minutes or until soft.

3.   Remove from the heat and let the soup cool slightly. Use an immersion blender to gently blend the soup inside the pot. If you don't have an immersion blender, transfer the soup to a blender and pulse until smooth. Taste and add a little more salt if necessary.

4.   Place the soup in the pot again over medium heat for about 2 or 3 minutes. Serve and accompany with toasted bread slices (optional).

Per serving: (1 medium bowl) Calories: 217; Total fat: 7.2g; Protein: 4.5g; Carbohydrates: 32g; Fiber: 4.3g

Pesto Pasta with Tofu

The classic Italian pesto pasta dish can be made very special by adding golden tofu cubes to increase the protein and make this rich dish a more complete one.

Servings: 2 | **Preparation:** 10 minutes | **Cooking:** 20 minutes

Ingredients

1 (6-ounce) block extra-firm tofu, drained
1 teaspoon olive oil
1 ⅓ tablespoons Bragg liquid aminos or coconut aminos
1 cup gluten-free pasta (preferably penne type)

To make the pesto:

½ cup fresh basil leaves
2 tablespoons walnuts
½ tablespoon extra virgin olive oil
1 tablespoon nutritional yeast
½ teaspoon sumac (optional)
¼ teaspoon salt

Preparation

1.   Cut the tofu block into small cubes and add them to a nonstick skillet over medium heat together with a teaspoon of oil and the Bragg liquid aminos or coconut aminos. Cook the tofu, turning it occasionally, until it is golden on the outside, 15 to 20 minutes.
2.   Add the pesto ingredients to a food processor and pulse several times (scraping the sides if necessary) until well combined. (You may need to add some water to help mix.) Taste and add a little more salt if necessary. Set aside.
3.   While the tofu is browning, place the pasta in a pot with boiling water and cook according to the package directions.
4.   Drain the pasta and return it to the pot. Pour the pesto sauce over the pasta and stir until well combined. Add the tofu and stir. Serve and enjoy.

Per serving: (½ of recipe) Calories: 277; Total fat: 9.8g; Protein: 14.2g; Carbohydrates: 30g; Fiber: 5g

Creamy Mushroom Pasta

A simple but tasty vegetarian recipe for gluten-free pasta with a rich and creamy mushroom sauce. Perfect for a light dinner during the week.

Servings: 2 | **Preparation:** 15 minutes | **Cooking:** 20 minutes

Ingredients

1 cup gluten-free pasta (rotini or fusilli type)
2 ¼ cups (5.5 ounces) mushrooms, sliced
½ tablespoon olive oil
½ leek (white part only), washed and chopped
½ tablespoon Bragg liquid aminos or coconut aminos
½ cup vegetable broth (you can also use water)
¼ cup unsweetened almond milk or other plant-based milk
1 tablespoon arrowroot flour or cornstarch (see note)
1 teaspoon fresh thyme, chopped (or ¼ teaspoon dried thyme)
½ teaspoon salt
1 tablespoon nutritional yeast (optional)
1 tablespoon fresh parsley, chopped (optional, for garnish)

Preparation

1.   Boil water in a medium saucepan and cook the pasta according to package directions.
2.   In a large, deep skillet over medium-high heat, add the olive oil and the leek and cook, stirring constantly, until the leek is golden brown, about 2 to 3 minutes.
3.   Add the mushrooms and thyme and cook until the mushrooms are soft, about 5 minutes. Add salt and cook for 1 more minute.
4.   Pour the vegetable broth (or water), Bragg liquid aminos, and nutritional yeast (if using). Mix well and bring to a boil.
5.   Dissolve the arrowroot flour or cornstarch in milk. Then pour the milk mixture into the pan and cook over low heat for about 5 minutes or until the sauce thickens.
6.   Once the sauce has thickened a little, add the pasta and mix well with the mushroom sauce. Serve and enjoy. Garnish with chopped parsley and serve!

Note

•   If you use cornstarch instead of arrowroot flour, I recommend that you use one that is NON-GMO (non-transgenic).

Per serving: (½ of recipe) Calories: 220; Total fat: 4.7g; Protein: 4.6g; Carbohydrates: 37.5g; Fiber: 2g

Veggie Tofu Stir-Fry

This is an excellent vegetarian alternative to Chinese-style stir-fry chicken or beef. It's perfect for lunch or dinner and ideal for serving with some white rice or cauliflower rice.

Servings: 1 | **Preparation:** 20 minutes | **Cooking:** 25 minutes

Ingredients

1 (3-ounce) block extra-firm tofu

¼ leek (white part only), washed and finely chopped

½ small carrot, peeled and cut into julienne or strips

½ cup broccoli florets, cut into pieces

¼ medium zucchini, sliced (optional)

2 teaspoons olive oil, divided

2 ½ tablespoons Bragg liquid aminos or coconut aminos

2 teaspoons sesame oil

½ teaspoon arrowroot flour or cornstarch (see note)

½ teaspoon ginger, grated

Preparation

1. Cut the tofu block into ½-inch cubes and place it in a nonstick skillet over medium heat along with a teaspoon of olive oil and a tablespoon of Bragg liquid aminos or coconut aminos. Cook the tofu, turning it occasionally, until it is golden on the outside, 15 to 20 minutes. Remove from the pan and set aside.

2. In a nonstick skillet over medium-high heat, add the leek, ginger, and remaining teaspoon of olive oil. Cook, stirring, until the leek is golden-brown, about 2 to 3 minutes.

3. Add the carrot, broccoli, and zucchini and cook, stirring constantly, until the vegetables are soft, about 5 to 7 minutes.

4. In a small bowl, mix the remaining Bragg liquid aminos or coconut aminos, sesame oil, and arrowroot flour or cornstarch. Pour over the sautéed vegetables and stir well. Cook over low heat, stirring occasionally, for an additional 2 or 3 minutes. Add the tofu and stir well. Serve and enjoy.

Note

• If you use cornstarch instead of arrowroot flour, I recommend that you use one that is NON-GMO (non-transgenic).

Per serving: (2 cups approx.) Calories: 132; Total fat: 7g; Protein: 10.4g; Carbohydrates: 7g; Fiber: 2.8g

Roasted Vegetable Burrito

A tasty and satisfying burrito loaded with nutritious vegetables such as sweet potatoes, zucchini, carrots, spinach, and avocado. It's perfect to take with you outside for lunch or dinner.

Servings: 2 | **Preparation:** 20 minutes | **Cooking:** 25 minutes

Ingredients

½ medium zucchini, chopped
½ medium carrot, peeled and chopped
½ small sweet potato, peeled and chopped into ½-inch pieces
1 tablespoon olive oil
1 cup fresh spinach
1 large egg + 1 egg white
½ cup chopped avocado or ⅓ cup guacamole (see recipe)
1 gluten-free flour tortilla
½ teaspoon salt

Preparation

1.   Preheat the oven to 425°F. Lightly grease the baking sheet with oil (preferably nonstick spray oil). Set aside.
2.   Place the zucchini, carrot, and sweet potato in a medium bowl and add ½ tablespoon of olive oil and ¼ teaspoon of salt. Mix the vegetables until they are well coated with the oil and salt.
3.   Spread the chopped vegetables evenly on the prepared baking sheet and bake for 20 to 25 minutes, until the vegetables are cooked and lightly browned.
4.   While the vegetables are in the oven, beat the egg, egg white, and remaining salt in a medium bowl.
5.   In a nonstick skillet over medium heat, add the remaining ½ tablespoon of oil and spinach. Cook, stirring occasionally, until the spinach is wilted, about 2 minutes.
6.   Pour the beaten eggs in the pan evenly over the spinach and cook, stirring constantly, for 1 or 2 minutes, until the egg is cooked.
7.   Heat the flour tortilla using the method of your choice (on an electric griddle, in a pan, or in the oven).
8.   Place the tortilla on a plate and add the roasted vegetables, scrambled eggs, and chopped avocado or guacamole (see recipe). Fold the sides of the tortilla and then roll it up to form a burrito.

Note

•   If you desire, you can substitute scrambled eggs for ½ cup of scrambled tofu, spinach for kale, and sweet potato for potato.

Per serving: (½ burrito) Calories: 209; Total fat: 8.4g; Protein: 9.6g; Carbs: 20g; Fiber: 6.8g

CHAPTER 8:SIDE DISH RECIPES

Sautéed Potatoes

These simple and tasty sautéed potatoes are perfect to accompany any meal and are an excellent alternative to French fries.

Servings: 2 | **Preparation:** 10 minutes | **Cooking:** 20 minutes

Ingredients

3 medium red or white potatoes
1 tablespoon olive oil
1 or 2 tablespoons fresh parsley, chopped
½ teaspoon dried rosemary
½ teaspoon salt

Preparation

1.   Peel and cut the potatoes into medium-sized pieces. Place the potatoes in a pot and cover them with water. Cook for about 15-18 minutes or until tender but still firm. (The cooking time depends on the size of the potatoes.) Drain the potatoes well.
2.   In a nonstick skillet over medium-high heat, add the oil and potatoes and cook, stirring constantly, until golden-brown, about 5 to 10 minutes.
3.   Once the potatoes are browned, add salt, rosemary, and parsley and mix well. Sauté the potatoes for another 30-60 seconds.
4.   Serve as an accompaniment to your main course.

Per serving: (½ of recipe) Calories: 245; Total fat: 3.6g; Protein: 4.3g; Carbs: 45g; Fiber: 5g

Simple Vegetable Rice

This recipe for vegetable rice is perfect for those days when you want to cook something out of the ordinary. Above all, it is simple and tastes delicious.

Servings: 2 | **Preparation:** 15 minutes | **Cooking:** 20 minutes

Ingredients

¾ cup white rice, rinsed and drained
1 ½ cups of vegetable broth (you can also use water)
½ medium carrot, diced
½ celery stalk, cut into pieces
½ cup zucchini, diced
⅛ leek stalk (white part only), finely chopped
1 tablespoon olive oil
½ teaspoon salt

Preparation

1.   Heat the oil in a nonstick skillet over medium heat. Add the carrot, celery, zucchini, and leek. Cook, stirring constantly, until the vegetables are tender, about 5 minutes. Set aside.
2.   In a medium saucepan, add the vegetable broth (or water) and salt and bring to a boil. Add the rice and let it boil until the water begins to dry.
3.   Once the water starts to dry (or when you don't see bubbles on the surface), reduce the heat to low and add the vegetables. Stir well and cook covered for 15 minutes.
4.   Uncover the rice and taste it. If you notice that it is still hard, stir it and cook covered for 5 or 10 more minutes. Remove the saucepan from the heat and stir the rice.
5.   Serve as an accompaniment to your main course.

Per serving: (1 cup approx.) Calories: 304; Total fat: 4g; Protein: 5.4g; Carbohydrates: 57g; Fiber: 3g

Turmeric Coconut Rice

This vibrant coconut-flavored rice not only is a side dish that tastes delicious but is also versatile enough to accompany any main course.

Servings: 2 | **Preparation:** 10 minutes | **Cooking:** 15 minutes

Ingredients

¾ cup white rice, rinsed and drained

½ cup canned coconut milk

1 cup of water or vegetable broth (see recipe)

½ teaspoon ground turmeric

1 teaspoon salt

¼ to ½ teaspoon fresh ginger, peeled and grated (optional)

Preparation

1.   In a medium saucepan, add the water or vegetable broth, turmeric, salt, and ginger (if using) and bring to a boil. Add the rice and coconut milk. Stir and let it boil until the water begins to evaporate.

2.   Once the water starts to evaporate (or when you don't see bubbles on the surface), reduce the heat to low. Stir and cook covered for 15-18 minutes. Remove the pot from the heat and stir the rice.

3.   Serve as an accompaniment to your main course.

Note

•   Turmeric is a very unpredictable spice, as it may cause stomach discomfort in some people. Therefore, it is recommended that you try the recipe and see how well you tolerate it.

Per serving: (1 cup approx.) Calories: 347; Total fat: 9g; Protein: 4.7g; Carbohydrates: 55g; Fiber: 2g

Roasted Butternut Squash

The slightly sweet taste and buttery texture of butternut squash combined with the flavor and aroma of fresh herbs make this side dish the ideal choice to accompany Christmas dinners or for a simple weekend dinner.

Servings: 2 | **Preparation:** 10 minutes | **Cooking:** 30 minutes

Ingredients

400g butternut squash (2 cups approx.)
1 ½ tablespoons fresh herbs (rosemary, thyme, oregano), chopped
1 tablespoon extra virgin olive oil
½ teaspoon salt
A pinch of ground cumin (optional)

Preparation

1.   Preheat the oven to 400°F. Grease a baking sheet with oil (preferably nonstick spray oil). Set aside.
2.   Remove the seeds and pulp from the center of the pumpkin. Peel it and cut it into 1-inch cubes.
3.   Place the pumpkin pieces onto a baking sheet. Drizzle with olive oil and sprinkle with the chopped fresh herbs and salt. Stir well to cover and spread the pumpkin pieces in a single layer.
4.   Bake in the preheated oven for 20 minutes. Remove from the oven and stir the pumpkin pieces. Return to the oven and bake about 10 more minutes.
5.   Serve as an accompaniment to your main course.

Per serving: (1 cup approx.) Calories: 110; Total fat: 3g; Protein: 1.8g; Carbohydrates: 14.5g; Fiber: 6.4g

Herb-Roasted Carrots

This simple side dish of roasted carrots with herbs is a healthy and delicious way to enjoy this root vegetable that is rich in antioxidants and beta-carotene.

Servings: 2 | **Preparation:** 10 minutes | **Cooking:** 30 minutes

Ingredients

2 medium carrots
½ tablespoon extra virgin olive oil
¼ teaspoon dried oregano
¼ teaspoon fresh thyme leaves, chopped
½ teaspoon salt
1 tablespoon parsley, finely chopped

Preparation

1.   Preheat the oven to 400°F. Grease a baking sheet with oil (preferably nonstick spray oil). Set aside.
2.   Peel the carrots and cut them lengthwise into 4 or 6 pieces (depending on the thickness), and then into pieces 2 inches long.
3.   Place the carrots in a large bowl and cover with the olive oil, salt, thyme, and oregano. Mix well.
4.   Spread the carrot pieces in a single uniform layer on the prepared baking sheet. Cover with foil and bake for 30 minutes. Uncover. If the carrots are not yet tender, lower the heat to 375° and return to the oven for 10 to 15 more minutes until they are tender.
5.   Add the parsley and stir slightly. Sprinkle with a little more salt if you want.
6.   Serve as an accompaniment to your main course.

Per serving: (½ of recipe) Calories: 55; Total fat: 3.5g; Protein: 1g; Carbohydrates: 4g; Fiber: 1.7g

Mashed Potatoes

A classic mashed potato recipe that, in addition to being simple, is quite easy to prepare and requires very few ingredients. It's an ideal accompaniment to tasty baked fish or grilled chicken.

Servings: 2 | **Preparation:** 10 minutes | **Cooking:** 25 minutes

Ingredients

2 medium red or white potatoes
¼ cup unsweetened almond milk or other plant-based milk
2 teaspoons extra virgin olive oil
½ teaspoon salt

Preparation

1. Peel and cut the potatoes into 4 pieces. Place the potatoes pieces in a pot and cover them with water. Add salt and bring to a boil. Cook covered for about 20-25 minutes until the potatoes are tender.
2. Once cooked, drain the potato pieces and place them in a medium bowl. Let the potatoes stand for a few minutes so that the extra water evaporates.
3. Mash the potatoes with a potato masher or fork. Add the olive oil and half of the milk to the bowl and mix until the puree has a smooth consistency. (If necessary, add more milk to the mashed potatoes until you reach the desired texture.)
4. Serve as an accompaniment to your main course.

Per serving: (½ of recipe) Calories: 196; Total fat: 5g; Protein: 3.4g; Carbohydrates: 31g; Fiber: 4.8g

Mashed Yuca

This delicious and soft mashed yuca (cassava) is the perfect alternative to typical mashed potatoes. Yuca is an energy-dense root vegetable with approximately twice the calories per serving as potatoes.

Servings: 2 | **Preparation:** 10 minutes | **Cooking:** 25 minutes

Ingredients

1 pound yuca (3 ½ cups approx.)
⅓ cup unsweetened almond milk or other plant-based milk
2 teaspoons extra virgin olive oil
1 teaspoon salt

Preparation

1.   Cut the ends of the yuca and remove the outer skin. Cut the yuca into pieces and place them in a pot. Cover the yuca pieces with water, add the salt, and bring to a boil over high heat. Cook covered for about 25-30 minutes until the yuca is soft.
2.   Once cooked, drain the yuca pieces and place them in a medium bowl. Remove the thick vein or fibrous stem from the center of the yuca pieces and mash them using a potato masher.
3.   Add the milk and olive oil. Mix until the puree has a smooth consistency. Add more milk to the yuca puree if it is too dry.
4.   Serve as an accompaniment to your main course.

Per serving: (½ of recipe) Calories: 416; Total fat: 5.5g; Protein: 3.3g; Carbohydrates: 84g; Fiber: 4.1g

Potato Wedges

These tasty baked potatoes are another excellent alternative to French fries. They're ideal to accompany a main course or you can enjoy them as a simple snack.

Servings: 2 | **Preparation:** 10 minutes | **Cooking:** 20-30 minutes

Ingredients

2 medium red or white potatoes
1 tablespoon extra virgin olive oil
1 teaspoon dried oregano
1 teaspoon dried thyme or rosemary
¼ teaspoon salt

Preparation

1.   Preheat the oven to 400°F.
2.   Wash the potatoes. Peel them and then cut them lengthwise in half in the form of wedges (at least 8 pieces).
3.   In a medium bowl, mix olive oil with oregano, thyme or rosemary, and salt. Add the potatoes to the bowl and stir until well combined.
4.   Place the potatoes on a baking sheet covered with parchment paper (or lightly grease the baking sheet) and bake for about 15 minutes.
5.   After 15 minutes, remove them from the oven and turn them on the other side. Bake for an additional 10-15 minutes or until they are golden-brown on the outside but soft on the inside when pricked. Watch them carefully so they don't burn.
6.   Serve as an accompaniment to your main course.

Note

•   You can use this same recipe to make wedges with other root vegetables such as sweet potatoes and parsnips.

Per serving: (½ of recipe) Calories: 191; Total fat: 4.6g; Protein: 3.2g; Carbohydrates: 31g; Fiber: 4.8g

CHAPTER 9:SNACK AND DESSERT RECIPES
Quick Snack Ideas

Before we start with snack and dessert recipes, I would like to give you some quick snack ideas that do not require much elaboration and that can be prepared using simple ingredients. The idea is that every time you are hungry, you can prepare something quick and easy, without having to wait a long time.

Chopped Fresh Fruits

A simple and healthy snack is a bowl of chopped fresh fruits. You can choose between fruits such as melon, watermelon, papaya, dragon fruit, and Bosc or Asian pears. Prepare approximately two cups of the fruit of your choice, or a combination of those mentioned above. A good combination of chopped fresh fruits is watermelon, cantaloupe, and papaya.

Toast or Rice Cakes

Gluten-free toast and puffed rice cakes are ideal with almond butter or mashed avocado. To prepare this simple snack, spread a tablespoon of almond butter or ⅓ cup of mashed avocado between one or two pieces of gluten-free toast or rice cakes.

Anti-Inflammatory Smoothies

Anti-inflammatory smoothies are another excellent snack, as, apart from being healthy and nutritious, they help fight inflammation in the stomach and within your body. To prepare them, use, as a base, a cup of almond milk or another plant-based milk (unsweetened) and half a cup of blueberries, strawberries, raspberries, or mixed berries. You can also add a very ripe banana (or other fruits), half a tablespoon of almond butter or a tablespoon of walnuts, or a tablespoon of pea or hemp protein powder. Add all the ingredients to a blender and blend until the mixture acquires a smooth consistency.

Baked Sweet Potato Fries

These tasty and slightly crispy baked sweet potatoes are another healthy alternative to typical French fries. Enjoy them as a snack or as an accompaniment to a main course.

Servings: 1 | **Preparation:** 10 minutes | **Cooking:** 25-30 minutes

Ingredients

1 medium sweet potato, peeled and cut into ¼-inch sticks
1 tablespoon extra virgin olive oil
½ teaspoon ground cumin
½ teaspoon dried oregano (optional)
½ teaspoon salt

Preparation

1.   Preheat the oven to 425°F.
2.   In a medium bowl, add the sweet potato sticks and cover with olive oil, cumin, and oregano (if using). Mix well.
3.   Place the sweet potato sticks in a single layer on a baking sheet covered with parchment paper (or lightly greased with a little oil). Make sure they are in a single layer and are not piled up.
4.   Bake for about 25-30 minutes, turning after the first 15 minutes, until the sweet potato sticks are golden-brown or slightly crispy on the outside and soft on the inside.
5.   Remove from the oven and let cool a few minutes. Sprinkle with salt.
6.   Serve with guacamole (optional, see recipe).

Note

•   For crispier sweet potatoes "fries", leave the sticks to soak in water for approximately 30 minutes (to remove excess starch). Then rinse and dry the sweet potato strips thoroughly absorbent paper towels and continue with step two of the preparation process.

Per serving: Calories: 162; Total fat: 6.9g; Protein: 2.3g; Carbohydrates: 19.7g; Fiber: 3.8g

Almond Flour Crackers

These tasty and easy to make almond flour crackers are great to snack on and take with you wherever you go.

Servings: 30-40 crackers | **Preparation:** 10 minutes | **Cooking:** 15 minutes

Ingredients

1 ¾ cups blanched almond flour, finely ground
1 large egg
1 tablespoon fresh rosemary, chopped (optional)
½ teaspoon salt

Preparation

1.   Preheat the oven to 350°F (175 degrees C).
2.   In a large bowl, mix the almond flour, salt, and rosemary (if using). Add the egg and mix well. Then, use your hands and mix until it forms a homogeneous dough.
3.   Place the dough between two large pieces of parchment paper. Use a rolling pin to roll the dough out to about 1/16 inch thick. Then remove the top piece of parchment paper.
4.   With a pizza cutter or a knife, cut the dough into 1-inch squares. If desired, sprinkle the crackers with salt. Transfer the bottom piece of parchment paper with the cut-out dough onto a baking sheet and bake for about 12 to 15 minutes, until the crackers are light golden brown.
5.   Remove from the oven and let cool for 10 minutes before gently separating them. Cool completely before serving.

Note

•   Leftovers may be stored in an airtight container in a cool, dry place for 3 to 5 days.

Per serving: (1 cracker approx.) Calories: 35; Total fat: 3.1g; Protein: 1.3g; Carbohydrates: 0.4g; Fiber: 0.6g

Baked Potato Chips

Satisfy your craving for something crispy with these delicious and healthy homemade baked potato chips.

Servings: 1 | **Preparation:** 30 minutes | **Cooking:** 15-20 minutes

Ingredients

1 medium potato
1 tablespoon extra virgin olive oil
½ teaspoon salt

Preparation

1.   Wash the potato, peel it, and cut it into thin slices (⅛ inch thick) with a mandoline slicer or knife.
2.   Soak the potato slices in cold water for about 20-30 minutes (to remove excess starch). Then rinse and completely dry the slices with absorbent paper towel or a clean cotton towel.
3.   Preheat the oven to 400°F.
4.   In a medium bowl, mix the potato slices with the olive oil. Then place them on a baking sheet covered with parchment paper (or grease with a little oil) and sprinkle with salt. Make sure they are in a single layer and not piled up.
5.   Bake for about 15-20 minutes or until crispy and lightly browned. (The time may vary depending on the oven and the thickness of the slices.) Watch them carefully to avoid burning.
6.   Remove from the oven and let cool a few minutes. Serve with guacamole (optional, see recipe).

Note

•   Soaking potato slices in cold water for at least 30 minutes is necessary to remove excess starch. The starch prevents moisture from escaping, which leaves more water in the potato and prevents the chips from getting crispy.

Per serving: Calories: 182; Total fat: 9g; Protein: 2.3g; Carbohydrates: 19g; Fiber: 3.8g

Tofu Nuggets

These amazing and healthy baked tofu nuggets are the perfect vegetarian alternative to traditional chicken nuggets. They're ideal to enjoy with a homemade sauce.

Servings: 2 | **Preparation:** 15 minutes | **Cooking:** 25 minutes

Ingredients

1 (12-ounce) block extra-firm tofu
½ cup gluten-free panko breadcrumbs
¼ cup gluten-free flour (any kind)
⅓ cup unsweetened almond milk or other plant-based milk
½ teaspoon salt
2 tablespoons nutritional yeast
½ teaspoon cumin
1 teaspoon Italian seasoning or dried parsley
Olive oil spray

Preparation

1.   Preheat the oven to 400°F.
2.   Remove the tofu from the package, drain it well, and cut it into approximately 10 or 12 slices.
3.   Place the tofu slices on a layer of absorbent paper towels (or a clean towel) and cover with another layer. Gently press down the tofu slices to absorb the extra water.
4.   In a medium bowl, combine the breadcrumbs, nutritional yeast, salt, cumin and Italian seasoning or dried parsley. Add the flour to a second bowl and add the milk to a third bowl.
5.   Dip each slice of tofu in the flour, then in the milk, and, finally, in the breadcrumb mixture. Repeat with the other slices.
6.   Place the tofu slices on a lightly greased baking sheet (or covered with parchment paper). Spray each slice with a thin layer of oil.
7.   Bake for 15 minutes. Turn on the other side and bake for about 10 minutes or until golden-brown. Watch them carefully so they don't burn.
8.   Remove from the oven and let cool slightly. Serve and enjoy.

Per serving: (5-6 nuggets approx.) Calories: 191; Total fat: 9g; Protein: 18g; Carbohydrates: 12g; Fiber: 1.4g

Blueberry Muffins

These delicious and fluffy blueberry muffins are a healthy alternative to traditional muffins, as they are low in fat and gluten- and dairy-free!

Servings: 12 muffins | **Preparation:** 10 minutes | **Cooking:** 25 minutes

Ingredients

3 cups gluten-free all-purpose flour
1 cup blueberries
1 ½ cups unsweetened almond milk or other plant-based milk
½ cup unsweetened applesauce
4 teaspoons baking powder
½ cup coconut sugar (see notes)
¼ teaspoon salt
1 teaspoon vanilla extract (optional)

Preparation

1. Preheat the oven to 400°F. Cover a 12-piece muffin pan with muffin liners or lightly grease each of the cups in the pan.
2. In a large bowl, combine the flour, baking powder, and salt.
3. In another medium bowl, mix the milk, applesauce, sugar, and vanilla (if using).
4. Slowly pour the wet ingredients into the bowl of the dry ingredients, stirring continuously. Mix until completely combined. Add the blueberries to the mixture and mix well.
5. Divide the mixture between the 12 cups of muffins and bake for 25-30 minutes or until the muffins are lightly browned on the top and when you insert a toothpick it comes out clean.
6. Remove from the oven and, after a few minutes, transfer the muffins to a cooling rack. Serve and enjoy.

Notes

•   If sugar is a problem for you, I recommend that you replace it with a sweetener such as maple syrup or monk fruit.
•   Muffins can be stored in an airtight container for 2 days at room temperature. However, it is better to keep them refrigerated (for up to 5 days).
•   If you want to add a little fat to your muffins, substitute about 2 or 4 tablespoons of the applesauce for the equivalent amount of coconut oil (preferably odorless coconut oil).

Per serving: (1 muffin) Calories: 154; Total fat: 1g; Protein: 1.6g; Carbohydrates: 34g; Fiber: 2g

Banana Bread

This delicious and amazing banana bread, apart from having an exquisite and sweet taste, is healthy and does not require eggs or dairy. It's ideal to enjoy as a dessert or at breakfast.

Servings: 10 slices | **Preparation:** 15 minutes | **Cooking:** 60 minutes

Ingredients

3 medium ripe bananas (1 ½ cups approx.)
1 ¾ cups gluten-free all-purpose flour (see notes)
¼ cup unsweetened almond milk or other plant-based milk
¼ cup melted coconut oil or applesauce (see notes)
¼ cup coconut sugar (optional, see notes)
¼ teaspoon salt
2 teaspoons baking powder
½ teaspoon baking soda
1 teaspoon vanilla extract (optional)

Preparation

1. Preheat the oven to 350°F. Lightly grease a 9x5-inch bread pan. Set aside.
2. Place the bananas in a medium bowl and mash them well with a potato masher or fork. Add the milk, coconut oil or applesauce, sugar, and vanilla (if using them). Mix until all the ingredients are incorporated into the mixture.
3. In another large bowl, combine the flour, baking powder, baking soda, and salt. Slowly pour the wet ingredients into the bowl of the dry ingredients, stirring continuously, and mix until completely combined.
4. Pour the mixture into the prepared bread pan and bake for 40 minutes.
5. After the first 40 minutes, take a look at the bread. If you notice the top is browning too fast, cover the bread pan with aluminum foil. Bake for an additional 10 or 15 minutes or until a toothpick inserted in the center of the bread comes out clean.
6. Remove from the oven and carefully remove the bread from the pan. Place it on a cooling rack and let it cool for at least 10 minutes before cutting it.

Notes

• If you want to create your own gluten-free all-purpose flour, you can make a mixture with 4 cups of rice flour, 1 cup of potato starch, ⅔ cup of tapioca flour, ⅓ cup of arrowroot powder, and 2 teaspoons of xanthan gum.
• If you want your bread to be low in fat, substitute unsweetened applesauce for coconut oil.
• If you use ripe-enough bananas, you may not have to add sugar to your banana bread. However, if you want a sweeter bread, you can add the amount of sugar indicated in the recipe. If sugar is a problem for you, you can substitute it for monk fruit or maple syrup.
• Store the bread in an airtight bag or container on the counter for up to 3 days or in the refrigerator for up to a week. Alternatively, you can keep the bread covered in the freezer as needed. You just have to defrost it overnight in the refrigerator and reheat it in a toaster oven or using the method of your choice.
• You can use this same recipe to make muffins. Simply pour the mixture into a muffin pan and bake for approximately 25 minutes.

Per serving: (1 slice) Calories: 174; Total fat: 6g; Protein: 2.5g; Carbohydrates: 27g; Fiber: 2.6g

Coconut Balls

These simple coconut balls are the perfect snack to take with you wherever you go, as they are small, healthy, and delicious.

Servings: 10 balls | **Preparation:** 15 minutes | **Cooking:** N/A

Ingredients

1 ¼ cups shredded coconut

⅓ cup almond flour

¼ cup maple syrup or honey

Preparation

1.   Place the almond flour, maple syrup, and 1 cup of shredded coconut in a food processor or blender and pulse until smooth. If the mixture is very sticky, add more shredded coconut or almond flour. If it is very hard, add more syrup or honey. The mixture must have the right consistency such that you can make balls with your hands.

2.   Pour the remaining shredded coconut into a small bowl. Make small balls with your hands (about 10 balls) and roll them in the shredded coconut. Add more shredded coconut if necessary.

3.   Place the balls on a plate and let cool in the refrigerator for at least an hour.

Per serving: (1 ball) Calories: 107; Total fat: 8.3g; Protein: 1.4g; Carbohydrates: 6.3g; Fiber: 2g

Pumpkin Custard

This creamy and rich pumpkin custard is a healthy alternative to custards based on milk and eggs. It's an ideal dessert to satisfy a craving for pumpkin pie.

Servings: 4 | **Preparation:** 10 minutes | **Cooking:** 5 minutes

Ingredients

1 ½ cups pumpkin puree (fresh or canned)
2 cups unsweetened almond milk or other plant-based milk
⅓ cup canned coconut milk
1 tablespoon unflavored gelatin or agar-agar powder
1 ½ teaspoons liquid stevia or 4 tablespoons coconut sugar
½ teaspoon cinnamon powder (optional, if tolerated)
1 teaspoon vanilla extract (optional)

Preparation

1.	In a medium bowl, add ⅓ cup of the milk and evenly sprinkle the gelatin on top. Let the gelatin hydrate for a few minutes until it gels.
2.	While the gelatin is hydrating, add the pumpkin puree, coconut milk, remaining milk, stevia, vanilla, and cinnamon (if tolerated) to a blender. Pulse until the mixture acquires a smooth consistency.
3.	Pour the mixture into a medium saucepan and cook over medium heat, stirring lightly, for about 5 minutes. (If it starts to boil, reduce the heat and continue stirring.) Turn off the heat.
4.	Once the gelatin gels, add it to the heated pumpkin mixture and mix well.
5.	Pour the pumpkin mixture into individual containers and let it cool for a while at room temperature. Then refrigerate for at least 2 hours or until firm.

Per serving: (1 cup approx.) Calories: 85; Total fat: 4.3g; Protein: 3.4g; Carbohydrates: 5.8g; Fiber: 2.6g

Banana Ice Cream

This soft, creamy, and naturally sweet banana ice cream is probably one of the easiest desserts you can make. Best of all, it does not require dairy milk or cream!

Servings: 1 | **Preparation:** 5 minutes | **Cooking:** N/A

Ingredients

2 ripe bananas, frozen and sliced
1-2 tablespoons unsweetened almond milk (more if necessary)

Preparation

1. Place the frozen bananas and milk in a food processor and pulse until the mixture has a consistency that resembles soft-serve ice cream. (Alternatively, you can use a high-speed blender.)
2. Serve immediately or freeze for at least 1 hour (if you want the ice cream to have a firmer consistency).

Flavorings

- Vanilla (base recipe + ½ teaspoon vanilla extract)
- "Chocolate" (base recipe + 1-2 tablespoons carob powder)
- Nut Butter (base recipe + 1 tablespoon almond or peanut butter)
- "Chocolate" Nut Butter (base recipe + 1 tablespoon carob powder + 1 tablespoon nut butter)
- Spirulina Ice Cream (base recipe + 1 teaspoon spirulina powder)
- Caramel Ice Cream (base recipe + 4-6 pitted Medjool dates + pinch of sea salt)
- Maple Walnut Ice Cream (base recipe + 1 tablespoon maple syrup + 1 tablespoon chopped walnuts)

Per serving: (2 bananas) Calories: 210; Total fat: 1g; Protein: 2.6g; Carbohydrates: 47g; Fiber: 6g

CHAPTER 10:EXTRA RECIPES

Homemade Gluten-Free Bread

An ideal recipe for bread lovers who prefer to avoid gluten and dairy. Excellent for sandwiches or toast, or spread with a little almond butter.

Servings: 15 slices | **Preparation:** 15 minutes | **Cooking:** 50 minutes

Ingredients

3 cups gluten-free all-purpose flour
1 ½ cups warm water or plant-based milk (approximately 110°F)
1 ¼ teaspoons xanthan gum (see notes)
2 ¼ teaspoons instant yeast
1 large egg
1 egg white
2 tablespoons olive oil
3 tablespoons coconut or brown sugar
1 teaspoon salt

Preparation

1. Grease a 9x5-inch bread pan. Set aside.
2. In a large bowl, combine the flour, xanthan gum, yeast, sugar, and salt.
3. In another bowl, combine the warm milk or water, eggs, and oil. Slowly pour the wet ingredients into the bowl of the dry ingredients, stirring continuously. Mix until they are completely combined. (You can use a hand mixer to mix all the ingredients.)
4. Pour the dough into the prepared bread pan and smooth the top. Cover the bread pan with a clean dishcloth or a piece of greased plastic wrap. Let the dough rise until it has doubled in size, about 1 hour.
5. When the dough has doubled in size, preheat the oven to 350°F. Remove the cloth or plastic wrap from the top of the bread pan.
6. Bake for 40-50 minutes or until the internal temperature reaches 190-200°F. Cover with foil after 30 minutes if you notice that the crust of the bread is beginning to brown too quickly.
7. Remove the bread from the oven and let cool for 2 minutes. Transfer the bread to a cooling rack and let it cool completely before cutting it.

Notes

• The amount of xanthan gum you add may vary depending on whether or not your gluten-free flour premix contains it. If the mix contains xanthan gum, add the amount indicated by the recipe. If not, add up to 3 teaspoons or the amount indicated by the manufacturer to make gluten-free bread.

• If you want to create your own gluten-free all-purpose flour, you can make a mixture with 4 cups of rice flour, 1 cup of potato starch, ⅔ cup of tapioca flour, ⅓ cup of arrowroot powder, and 2 teaspoons of xanthan gum.

• Store the bread in an airtight bag or container on the counter for up to 3 days. Alternatively, you can refrigerate or freeze as needed, though keep in mind that gluten-free bread will dry quickly once cooled. You can heat it in a toaster oven or using the method you prefer to help soften it again.

Per serving: (1 slice) Calories: 114; Total fat: 3g; Protein: 3.1g; Carbohydrates: 18g; Fiber: 2g

Homemade Non-Dairy Milk

An easy and simple recipe for making a variety of delicious, creamy, and healthy plant-based "milks" that are free of additives and preservatives. It's perfect to use in your favorite recipes or just to drink directly.

Servings: 3-4 cups | **Preparation:** 15 minutes | **Cooking:** N/A

Ingredients

1 cup nuts or raw seeds of your choice (almonds, cashews, hemp or sunflower seeds, etc.)
3 or 4 cups filtered or purified water
A pinch of salt

Optional add-ins:

2 tablespoons maple syrup or ¼ teaspoon liquid stevia
1 teaspoon vanilla extract

Preparation

1.   Place the nuts or seeds in a medium bowl and cover with 2-3 cups of water. Cover the bowl with a cloth and let it soak overnight at room temperature. Cashews require only 2-3 hours of soaking, while Brazil nuts, hemp seeds, flaxseeds, and shredded coconut do not require soaking. If you use flaxseeds, use only ⅓ cup.
2.   Discard the soaking water and rinse the nuts or seeds thoroughly through a strainer.
3.   Place the nuts or seeds in a blender and add 3-4 cups of filtered or purified water. Pulse until smooth.
4.   Pour the mixture into a nut milk bag (or 2 layers of cheesecloth) and squeeze into a large bowl until all the liquid is extracted.
5.   Add the sweetener of your choice and vanilla (if using) and mix well. Transfer to a glass jar or airtight container with a lid and store the milk in the refrigerator for up to 4 days.

Notes

•   You can use this same recipe to make oat, rice, or coconut milk. For that, I recommend that you use 1 cup of oats or 2 cups of unsweetened shredded coconut for every 3-4 cups of filtered water. Heat the water to make coconut milk.
•   Be sure to shake the milk well before using it.

Homemade Vegetable Broth

This simple homemade vegetable broth is a great alternative to broths full of irritating ingredients sold in supermarkets. It's an excellent way to add flavor to soups, stews, or any dish that calls for it.

Servings: 6 cups approx. | **Preparation:** 15 minutes | **Cooking:** 60 minutes

Ingredients

2 medium carrots, peeled and chopped
2 celery stalks, chopped
1 leek (white part only), rinsed and chopped
1 fennel bulb, chopped (see notes)
2 bay leaves
3 sprigs fresh parsley
3 sprigs fresh thyme or 1 teaspoon dried thyme
8 cups filtered water

Preparation

1.   Place all the ingredients in a large pot and bring to a boil over high heat.
2.   Once it starts to boil, reduce the heat to low and cover with a lid. Let the vegetable broth simmer for at least 1 hour.
3.   Remove from heat and pour the broth through a fine-mesh strainer into a large bowl or pot. Discard the vegetables.
4.   Let the broth cool for about half an hour and then separate into glass containers for storage.
5.   Refrigerate the broth for up to a week or freeze it indefinitely.

Note

•   If you can't find the fennel bulb, you can skip it. It is recommended that you shake or stir the vegetable broth before using it.

Simple Guacamole

This simple and tasty guacamole is super easy to make and requires few ingredients. It's an ideal accompaniment for potato chips or baked sweet potato fries.

Servings: 1 | **Preparation:** 5 minutes | **Cooking:** N/A

Ingredients

½ cup ripe avocado, peeled, pitted, and chopped

1 tablespoon fresh cilantro, chopped

¼ teaspoon salt

¼ teaspoon sumac or grated lemon zest

A pinch of ground cumin

Preparation

1.   In a small bowl, add all the ingredients and puree with a masher or fork.

Note

•   If, after preparing this guacamole, you decide to save it for later, I recommend that you place plastic wrap directly on it to prevent the avocado from oxidizing.

Per serving: (½ cup) Calories: 90; Total fat: 7.5g; Protein: 1.7g; Carbohydrates: 1.6g; Fiber: 4.2g

Basil Walnut Pesto

This recipe for basil and walnut pesto is packed with healthy fats and is delicious in almost everything. It's ideal for pasta or spread on sandwiches or a simple piece of bread.

Servings: ½ cup | **Preparation:** 10 minutes | **Cooking:** N/A

Ingredients

½ cup fresh basil leaves

¼ cup walnuts

1 or 2 tablespoons extra virgin olive oil

1 tablespoon nutritional yeast

½ teaspoon sumac or grated lemon zest

½ teaspoon salt

Preparation

1.   In a food processor or blender, add all the ingredients and pulse for about 30 or 60 seconds (scraping the sides if necessary) until combined. Depending on whether you use a blender or a food processor, you may need to add a little water to help with the mixing.

Per serving: (2 tablespoons approx.) Calories: 77; Total fat: 7.5g; Protein: 1.8g; Carbohydrates: 1g; Fiber: 1g

Black Olive Tapenade

Tapenade is a rich and savory olive-based Mediterranean spread that, while it doesn't look very appetizing, has an exquisite flavor and is delicious on crackers or toast.

Servings: ½ cup | **Preparation:** 15 minutes | **Cooking:** N/A

Ingredients

½ cup black olives, chopped and pitted (see notes)
½ anchovy fillet, finely chopped
2 tablespoons fresh basil, chopped
1 teaspoon fresh thyme, chopped
1 tablespoon extra virgin olive oil

Preparation

1.   Place the olives, anchovy, basil, and thyme in a food processor and pulse until the ingredients are crushed well. (Alternatively, place the ingredients in a mortar and pestle, and then tap and crush with the pestle until the ingredients have been reduced to a thick paste.)
2.   While the food processor is running, gradually add olive oil until everything is well combined and a paste forms.
3.   Serve on gluten-free toast or crackers, or transfer to an airtight container and store in the refrigerator.

Notes

•   To prepare this tapenade, it is recommendable to use Kalamata olives, which have a more complex flavor than the generic black olives sold in supermarkets.
•   When storing the tapenade, pour a little olive oil over the surface of the tapenade to avoid oxidation.

Per serving: (2 tablespoons approx.) Calories: 54; Total fat: 5.5g; Protein: 1g; Carbohydrates: 1g; Fiber: 1g

Mushroom Sauce

This rich and creamy mushroom sauce is ideal over your favorite pasta. It's also versatile enough to be poured over some delicious meatballs or grilled chicken.

Servings: 1 | **Preparation:** 15 minutes | **Cooking:** 15 minutes

Ingredients

2 ¼ cups (5.5 ounces) mushrooms, sliced
½ tablespoon olive oil
½ leek (white part only), chopped
½ tablespoon Bragg liquid aminos or coconut aminos
½ cup vegetable broth (you can also use water)
¼ cup unsweetened almond milk or other plant-based milk
1 tablespoon arrowroot flour or cornstarch (see note)
1 teaspoon fresh thyme, chopped (or ¼ teaspoon dried thyme)
1 tablespoon nutritional yeast (optional)
½ teaspoon salt

Preparation

1.   In a large, deep skillet over medium-high heat, add the olive oil and leek. Cook, stirring constantly, until the leek is golden brown, about 2 to 3 minutes.
2.   Add the mushrooms and thyme. Cook until the mushrooms are soft, about 5 minutes. Add salt and cook for 1 more minute.
3.   Pour the vegetable broth (or water) and add the Bragg liquid aminos and nutritional yeast (if using). Mix well and bring to a boil.
4.   Dissolve the arrowroot flour or cornstarch in milk. Pour the milk mixture into the pan and cook over medium-low heat for about 5 minutes or until the sauce thickens.

Note

•   If you use cornstarch instead of arrowroot flour, I recommend that you use one that is NON-GMO (non-transgenic).

Per serving: (½ of recipe) Calories: 70; Total fat: 3g; Protein: 3g; Carbohydrates: 7.4g; Fiber: 1.3g

Stir-Fry Sauces

These delicious and healthy stir-fry sauces are the perfect alternative to the typical stir-fry sauces full of irritating ingredients sold in supermarkets.

Servings: ⅓ cup approx. | **Preparation:** 5 minutes | **Cooking:** N/A

Ingredients for recipe #1

¼ cup coconut aminos or Bragg liquid aminos

2 tablespoons sesame oil

½ tablespoon arrowroot flour or cornstarch (see notes)

Ingredients for recipe #2

2 tablespoons coconut aminos or Bragg liquid aminos

¼ cup vegetable broth (see recipe)

1 teaspoon arrowroot flour or cornstarch (see notes)

½ teaspoon fish sauce (see notes)

¼ teaspoon ground ginger

Preparation

1.   To make any of the above recipes for stir-fry sauces, simply mix all the ingredients.

Notes

•   If you use cornstarch instead of arrowroot flour, I recommend that you use one that is NON-GMO (non-transgenic).

•   You can skip the fish sauce from the second recipe if you are going to prepare a vegetarian stir-fry.

•   If you want a touch of sweetness to your stir-fry sauce, you can add a dash of maple syrup.

Salad Dressings

These simple salad dressing recipes are an excellent alternative to the typical store-bought salad dressings, which are usually loaded with additives and irritating ingredients that cause inflammation and slow the healing process. Use these simple and healthy dressings to give your salads the touch of flavor they need.

Simple Herb Dressing

¼ teaspoon fresh parsley, finely chopped
¼ teaspoon fresh oregano, finely chopped
¼ teaspoon fresh basil, finely chopped
1 tablespoon extra virgin olive oil
A pinch of salt
A pinch of sumac (optional)

In a small cup, mix all the dressing ingredients. Pour over the salad and enjoy.

Papaya Dressing

½ cup papaya, chopped
1 tablespoon extra virgin olive oil
½ teaspoon sumac or grated lemon zest
1 tablespoon fresh thyme, chopped
¼ teaspoon salt
1 or 2 tablespoons water (optional, if necessary)

In a food processor or blender, add all the ingredients (except water) and pulse until smooth. Taste and add more salt if necessary. Pour the dressing over the salad and enjoy.

Carrot Ginger Dressing

½ medium carrot, peeled and chopped
1 ¼ tablespoons extra virgin olive oil
¼ tablespoon fresh ginger, peeled and chopped
2 teaspoons maple syrup or honey
½ teaspoon toasted sesame oil
¼ teaspoon sumac or grated lemon zest
¼ teaspoon salt
1 or 2 tablespoons of water (optional, if necessary)

In a food processor or blender, add all the ingredients (except water) and pulse until smooth. Dilute with water if necessary. Pour the dressing over the salad and enjoy.

Peanut Dressing

2 tablespoons creamy peanut butter
¼ teaspoon ground ginger
1 tablespoon honey or maple syrup
2 tablespoons water
1 tablespoon Bragg liquid aminos or coconut aminos
2 pinches of sumac

In a small bowl, mix all the dressing ingredients. Pour over the salad and enjoy.

Creamy Avocado Dressing

¼ cup avocado
1 tablespoons olive oil
2 tablespoons water or more to give consistency
1 teaspoon plain non-dairy yogurt (optional)
1 tablespoon cilantro, basil, or parsley
½ teaspoon sumac or grated lime zest
¼ teaspoon salt

In a food processor, combine all the ingredients and pulse until smooth. Dilute with more water if necessary. Pour the dressing over the salad and enjoy.

CPSIA information can be obtained
at www.ICGtesting.com
Printed in the USA
BVHW051704030122
625349BV00015B/390